HEALING
Gourmet
Eat to Boost
Fertility

HEALING
Gourmet®
Eat to Boost
Fertility

THE EDITORS OF HEALING GOURMET WITH

Victoria Rand, M.D.,

Melissa Ohlson, M.S., RD, and Bev Shaffer

McGraw·Hill

New York   Chicago   San Francisco   Lisbon   London   Madrid   Mexico City
Milan   New Delhi   San Juan   Seoul   Singapore   Sydney   Toronto

The *McGraw·Hill* Companies

Library of Congress Cataloging-in-Publication Data

Healing gourmet, eat to boost fertility / with Victoria Rand, Melissa Ohlson, and Bev Shaffer.
    p.   cm.
Includes bibliographical references and index.
ISBN 0-07-146199-X (alk. paper)
    1. Infertility, Female—Diet therapy—Popular works.   2. Infertility, Female—Diet therapy—Recipes.   3. Infertility, Female—Nutritional aspects—Popular works.   4. Infertility, Male—Nutritional aspects—Popular works.   5. Infertility—Nutritional aspects—Popular works.   I. Ohlson, Melissa. II. Shaffer, Bev, 1951–.   III. Healing gourmet.   IV. Title.

RG201.R36   2006
618.1'780654—dc22   2005017027

1 2 3 4 5 6 7 8 9 0   FGR/FGR   0 9 8 7 6 5

ISBN 0-07-146199-X

Interior design by Monica Baziuk

McGraw-Hill books are available at special quantity discounts to use as premiums and sales promotions, or for use in corporate training programs. For more information, please write to the Director of Special Sales, Professional Publishing, McGraw-Hill, Two Penn Plaza, New York, NY 10121-2298. Or contact your local bookstore.

This book is printed on acid-free paper.

*To future moms and dads: it's a tough job
but somebody's gotta "do it."*

Contents

Acknowledgments

THIS BOOK IS brought to you with the assistance and knowledge of medical, culinary, and nutrition experts from across the nation, as well as the diligent work of countless scientists worldwide that help us to translate "research to recipes" in our mission to educate on the link between diet and disease. Healing Gourmet would like to thank the following people for their contribution.

A very special thanks to our book editor, Natasha Graf, for her attention to detail and function as catalyst for many of the concepts presented in the book, and to our project editor, Nancy Hall, for her excellent work in the final editing of the manuscript.

Our medical, nutrition, and culinary editors: Thanks to Dr. Victoria Rand for her thorough review and guidance; to Melissa Ohlson for her speedy and meticulous work on recipe analysis, meal planning, and nutritional review; and Bev Shaffer for her culinary expertise to ensure our recipes deliver as much taste as they do health. A special thanks to Chef Paul Jones for running the Healing Gourmet test kitchen.

Our publisher: Thanks to McGraw-Hill for their commitment to delivering high-quality information to the public, including many of the educational textbooks that spurred the development of this company.

Our affiliations: Thanks to the fine institutions that bring us these editors, including the University of California and the Cleveland Clinic Foundation.

Our associates and family: Thanks to Guy Gelin and our friends and families for their continuing support of the Healing Gourmet project.

Introduction

HEALING GOURMET® BEGAN with a mission to educate people on the link between diet and disease. As part of a series, this book is meant to provide useful information on eating to boost fertility through sound nutritional principles. We bring the "clinic" together with the "kitchen," to help you deliciously make the most of your health through the latest discoveries. Quite simply, Healing Gourmet translates research to recipes, making your kitchen a healing haven.

In this book, we will show you how your diet can help to boost your fertility and manage syndromes associated with conception issues and pregnancy. Chapters 1 and 2 focus on the basic principles of fertility and the barriers to conception including PCOS, insulin resistance, and other hormonal factors. In Chapters 3 and 4, we give you the skinny on fat and carbohydrates and how they affect your hormones; and we introduce you to your pregnancy-boosting arsenal of phytonutrients and antioxidants. We devote Chapter 5 to the men and provide specific nutrients found to boost sperm count and the foods you can find them in. In Chapters 6 and 7 we deliver the delicious foods to be fruitful, help you prepare for pregnancy with optimal prenatal nutrition, and show you how to combat common deficiencies.

Of course, we'll help you to sleuth out the healthiest products at the grocery in Chapter 8, plan your menus for optimal fertility in Chapter 9, and give you fifty great recipes to get you started in Chapter 10. Don't forget to visit our website, healing gourmet.com, to find the latest research and more pregnancy-boosting recipes!

Important disclaimer: The information in this book cannot replace the advice of your physician or health-care team. Always consult with your doctor before making any changes in diet.

Letter from the Editor

CAN SOMETHING AS delicious as Sesame Salmon Roulades really help to balance blood sugar, reduce the risk of PCOS, and enhance fertility? Or can a recipe for a Father-to-Be Smoothie help boost sperm count? These are just a couple of the questions we set out to answer nearly five years ago with the creation of our company. Dedicated solely to helping the public make better choices about the foods to eat to prevent and mitigate nutrition-related diseases, Healing Gourmet brings you sound, scientific evidence and practical solutions to help you take control of your health.

Our recipe for health is simple. First, we take a disease-fighting dose of research, collected from the National Library of Medicine on your favorite foods, compounds in foods, and their effects on disease. Right at this very moment, scientists are hard at work analyzing nutrients in foods for their beneficial effects on blood sugar and hormones, their cholesterol-lowering capacity, and their cancer-fighting action. Other researchers are poring over data from population studies to give us clues to why disease rates are lower in other countries where their diets differ greatly from those in the United States. Together, this research in the new nutritional frontier acts as the foundation—the first ingredient—in a health-promoting mix. To help us in this research, we are extremely fortunate to have the assistance of Victoria Rand, M.D. Dr. Rand is a volunteer professor at the University of California at San Francisco and is board certified in internal medicine with training in acupuncture, herbal medicine, and other complementary therapies. The next step in our recipe for health is incorporating these scientific findings with culinary finesse to whip up mouthwatering recipes and easy-to-use meal plans that help you make the most of the latest nutritional breakthroughs. For this task, we are also lucky to have the expertise and nutritional analysis of Melissa Ohlson, M.S., RD—the nutrition projects coordinator, Preventive Cardiology and Rehabilitation at the Cleveland Clinic Heart Center—and the culinary expertise of Bev Shaffer, culinary expert of "Cooking for Your Heart" Program in association with the Cleveland Clinic Foundation. More on these amazing contributors is listed in the next section.

Don't forget to visit us on the Web at healinggourmet.com and look for us on television this fall debuting on the Healthy Living Channel. Enjoy these books in good health and *eat your medicine*!

—KELLEY LUNSFORD
Editor-in-Chief
Chairman, President, and CEO

About the Contributors

Medical Editor

Victoria Rand, M.D., is an assistant clinical professor in the Department of Medicine at the University of California at San Francisco. She currently practices at California Pacific Medical Center in San Francisco and she also has a private acupuncture practice. Dr. Rand has lectured widely and received her M.D. with distinction at Cornell University Medical College.

Nutrition Editor

Melissa Ohlson, M.S., RD, is the nutrition projects coordinator, Preventive Cardiology and Rehabilitation at the Cleveland Clinic Heart Center. Her broad scope of work includes medical nutrition therapy, speaking on nutrition and health coordination of nutrition activities at the clinic, development of online nutrition programs, and coordination of the "Cooking for Your Heart" culinary program series. Melissa is also a personal trainer and a nutrition consultant.

Culinary Editor

Bev Shaffer is the director of the cooking school and bakery operations at the Mustard Seed Market and Café in Cleveland, Ohio, and is the culinary expert of "Cooking for Your Heart" at the Section of Cardiology and Rehabilitation at the Cleveland Clinic Foundation. Her extensive work with this unique outreach program incorporates sound nutrition principles with delicious flavors, educating the public through culinary classes and tastings.

Understanding Fertility

Bringing a child into the world is one of life's little miracles. Unfortunately for some, achieving conception seems like a miracle in itself. You are not alone. In fact, infertility affects about 6.1 million Americans, or 10 percent of the reproductive age population, according to the American Society for Reproductive Medicine. The good news is that with modern science and technology, we have a better understanding of the reproductive process and how we can boost fertility and achieve pregnancy through a healthy lifestyle and sometimes the helping hand of reproductive specialists. While Father Time may not be on your side, Mother Nature is. In this book, we'll explore how nutrition can help you boost fertility and promote a successful pregnancy.

Pregnancy is the result of a chain of events. A woman must release an egg from one of her ovaries (known as *ovulation*), the egg must travel through the fallopian tube toward her uterus (or womb), and a man's sperm must join with (or fertilize) the egg along the way. The fertilized egg must then become attached to the inside of the uterus. While this may seem simple, in fact many things can happen to prevent pregnancy from occurring.

Infertility is usually defined as not being able to get pregnant despite trying for one year or not being able to carry a pregnancy to full term. We know that nutrition can impact fertility and reproduction. For women, whether or not you choose to have children, diet and lifestyle choices made during childbearing years can have long-term effects on fertility. However, it is a myth that infertility is always a "woman's problem." About one-third of infertility cases are due to problems with the man (male factors) and one-third are due to problems with the woman (female factors). The remaining third of cases are due to a combination of male and female factors or to unknown causes. In this chapter, we will help you understand the basic risk factors and causes of infertility in both men and women, ways to chart your fertility pattern, and some of the basic tests and medical treatments for infertility.

Causes of Female Infertility

Problems with ovulation (*ovulatory infertility*) account for most infertility in women, and research is emerging on how dietary measures can improve fertility by promoting ovulation, which we will focus on throughout the book. While a number of causes can lead to infertility in women, this book is going to focus mainly on the medical conditions where nutritional factors can help to alleviate fertility problems. However, let's take a quick look at some of these medical conditions and how they affect fertility.

Endometriosis

Experts estimate that up to one in ten American women of childbearing age have endometriosis, and of those with the condition, 30 to 40 percent are infertile. Endometriosis occurs when the tissue that makes up the lining of the uterus (or *endometrium*) grows outside of the uterus. Most commonly, this tissue is implanted on the ovaries or the lining of the abdomen near the uterus, fallopian tubes, and ovaries. Hormonal cycles cause the tissue to grow, shed, and bleed in sync with the lining of the uterus each month, which can lead to scarring and inflammation. Pelvic pain and infertility are common, and recent research shows diet may have an effect on women with endometriosis. (We will discuss this research in more detail in Chapter 2.)

Ovulation Disorders

About 25 percent of female infertility is caused by ovulation disorders. Even slight irregularities in the hormone system can affect ovulation. When the part of the brain that regulates ovulation (the *hypothalamic-pituitary axis*) is disrupted, deficiencies in luteinizing hormone (LH) and follicle-stimulating hormone (FSH) can occur, reducing chances of conception. Specific causes of hypothalamic-pituitary disorders include injury to the hypothalamus or pituitary gland, pituitary tumors, excessive exercise, and anorexia nervosa. In Chapters 2 and 3, we will discuss how lifestyle factors including weight, body mass index (BMI), and diet affect ovulation.

Polycystic Ovary Syndrome (PCOS)

PCOS is the most common form of infertility related to a lack of ovulation (*anovulatory infertility*). In PCOS, there is an increased risk of insulin resistance, diabetes, metabolic syndrome, cardiovascular disease, and other inflammatory disorders. PCOS causes an increase in the production of androgens (male-type hormones); and in women with increased body mass, elevated androgen production may come from stimulation by higher levels of insulin. In lean women, the elevated levels of androgen may be caused by a higher ratio of LH. Lack of menstruation (*amenorrhea*) or infrequent menses (*oligomenorrhea*) are common symptoms in women with PCOS, and a lack of ovulation may lead to mild enlargement of the ovaries. Without ovulation, the hormone progesterone isn't produced and estrogen levels remain constant. Elevated levels of androgen may cause increased dark or thick hair on the chin, upper lip, or lower abdomen as well as acne and oily skin.

Research is emerging on how diet and lifestyle can benefit PCOS and promote fertility. We will discuss how balancing hormones, reducing inflammation, and optimizing your weight benefit PCOS in Chapter 2, as well as the specific dietary recommendations to help you accomplish this in Chapters 3, 4, and 5.

Other Factors

A number of other factors can lead to infertility in women including use of certain medications (contraceptives) or disorders of the thyroid, and cancers and cancer treatments—including radiation and chemotherapy. In addition, diseases such as Cushing's disease, sickle cell anemia, HIV/AIDS, kidney disease, and diabetes can also affect fertility. Other factors of infertility include:

❖ **Fallopian tube damage or blockage.** This condition usually results from inflammation of the fallopian tube (*salpingitis*). Sexually transmitted diseases (STDs), such as chlamydia, are the most common cause. Tubal inflammation may go unnoticed or cause pain and fever, and the resulting scarring prevents a fertilized egg to make its way from the fallopian tube to implant in the uterus, causing an *ectopic pregnancy*. The risk of ectopic pregnancy increases with each occurrence of tubal infection.

❖ **Elevated prolactin (*hyperprolactinemia*).** Prolactin stimulates breast milk production and high levels in women who aren't pregnant or nursing may affect ovulation. A sign of elevated prolactin is milk flow unrelated to pregnancy or nursing. Elevated prolactin levels may also indicate the presence of a pituitary tumor.

❖ **Early menopause (premature ovarian failure).** The absence of menstruation, and the early depletion of ovarian follicles before age thirty-five, is a subject that receives little attention, and yet, around one in one hundred women experience these symptoms of early menopause.

❖ **Benign fibroid tumors.** Common among women in their thirties, fibroids are benign tumors in the wall of the uterus. Sometimes they may cause infertility by interfering with the contour of the uterine cavity, blocking the fallopian tubes or preventing implantation.

❖ **Pelvic adhesions.** These are bands of scar tissue that bind organs after pelvic infection, appendicitis, or abdominal or pelvic surgery, which may limit the functioning of the ovaries and fallopian tubes and impair fertility.

Risk Factors for Female Infertility

Irregular menstrual periods and conditions that cause pain during menstruation or intercourse may signal infertility. These are many of the risk factors for female infertility. Age is the strongest predictor of female fertility, with a steady decline after age thirty-two. The risk of miscarriage also increases with a woman's age. Chromosomal abnormalities occur in the eggs as they age, which may also contribute to infertility. Older women are also more likely to have health problems that may interfere with fertility.

Women who smoke tobacco may reduce their chances of becoming pregnant, decrease the possible benefit of fertility treatment, and have a higher risk of miscarriages. There's also no certain level of safe alcohol use during conception or pregnancy.

Extremes in body mass—either too high (body mass index, or BMI, of greater than 25) or too low (BMI of lower than 20)—may affect ovulation and increase the risk of infertility. However, research shows that 25 percent of ovulatory infertility is related to being overweight where only 12 percent can be attributed to being underweight. Among American women, infertility often is due to a sedentary lifestyle and being overweight, and is strongly related with PCOS and other hormonal factors affecting fertility.

In addition, being underweight can also affect your ability to conceive. Women at risk include those with eating disorders, such as anorexia nervosa or bulimia, and women on a very low-calorie or restrictive diet that may not provide adequate calories or nutrients to support conception and pregnancy. Strict vegetarians also may experience infertility problems and must find ways to get important nutrients such as vitamin B_{12}, zinc, iron, and folic acid. Extreme athletes who exercise very intensely are more prone to menstrual irregularities and infertility.

Causes of Infertility in Men

Infertility in men is often caused by problems with making sperm or getting the sperm to reach the egg successfully. Problems with sperm may exist from birth or develop later in life because of illness or injury. Some men produce no sperm or produce too few sperm.

Sperm Abnormalities

More than 90 percent of male infertility causes are due to sperm abnormalities that include the following.

❖ **Impaired shape (*morphology*) and movement (*motility*) of sperm.** Sperm must be properly shaped and able to move rapidly and accurately toward the egg for fertilization to occur.

❖ **Low sperm concentration.** Fewer than 13.5 million sperm per milliliter of semen indicates low sperm concentration. Fertility is defined as 48 million sperm per milliliter of semen.

❖ **Absent sperm production in testicles.** Although very rare, the complete failure of the testicles to produce sperm occurs in less than 5 percent of infertile men.

❖ **Varicocele.** Essentially a varicose vein in the scrotum, varicoceles prevent normal cooling of the testicle and raise testicular temperature, preventing sperm from surviving.

✤ **Undescended testicle.** This condition occurs when one or both testicles fail to descend from the abdomen into the scrotum during fetal development, resulting in mild to severely impaired sperm production. Also, because the testicles are exposed to the higher degree of internal body heat, sperm production may be affected.

✤ **Testosterone deficiency (*male hypogonadism*).** Having too little testosterone either comes from testicular disorders or a condition affecting the hypothalamus or pituitary glands in the brain that produce the hormones that control the testicles.

✤ **Klinefelter's syndrome.** A genetic disorder of the sex chromosomes, this syndrome causes a man to have two X chromosomes and one Y chromosome instead of one X and one Y. Klinefelter's syndrome results in abnormal development of the testicles, low or absent sperm production, and reduced testosterone production.

✤ **Infections.** A number of infections may temporarily affect sperm motility, including sexually transmitted diseases (STDs) such as chlamydia and gonorrhea, which cause scarring and block sperm passage. Mycoplasma; mumps; and infection of the prostate, urethra, or epididymis may also alter sperm motility.

✤ **Genetics.** When sperm concentration is fewer than five million per milliliter of semen, genetic causes may be involved. Blood testing can reveal whether there are subtle changes in the Y chromosome affecting fertility.

Other Factors

In addition, getting the sperm from the penis into the vagina is also to blame for infertility. Problems that affect this include the following.

✤ **Sexual issues.** Problems with sexual intercourse or technique may affect fertility. Erectile dysfunction, premature ejaculation, painful intercourse, as well as psychological or relationship problems can contribute to infertility. Sexual lubricants can also be toxic to sperm and impair fertility.

❖ **Blockage of the ejaculatory ducts or epididymis.** In some cases, men are born with blockage of the part of the testicle that contains sperm (*epididymis*) or ejaculatory ducts. Similarly, about 2 percent of men who seek treatment for infertility lack the tubes that carry sperm (*vas deferens*).

❖ **Retrograde ejaculation.** Instead of semen emerging through the penis during orgasm, it enters the bladder in retrograde ejaculation. Diabetes; bladder, prostate, or urethral surgery; and the use of psychiatric or antihypertensive drugs are causes of this problem.

❖ **Absence of semen (*ejaculate*).** The absence of ejaculate can rarely occur in men with specific disease or spinal cord injuries or diseases.

❖ **Misplaced urinary opening (*hypospadias*).** Having the urinary opening to be abnormally located on the underside of the penis can prevent sperm from reaching the cervix.

❖ **Antisperm antibodies.** Presence of antibodies that target sperm and weaken or disable them affects the likelihood of conception and usually occurs after surgical blockage of part of the vas deferens for male sterilization *(vasectomy)*.

❖ **Cystic fibrosis.** Men with this genetic disorder often have missing or obstructed vas deferens (the tubes that carry sperm).

Risk Factors for Male Infertility

Most men with infertility experience no signs or symptoms, although some men with hormonal changes may notice alterations in their voice or pattern of hair growth, an enlargement of their breasts, or difficulty with sexual function. Many of the risk factors for male and female infertility are the same. A gradual decline in fertility is common in men older than thirty-five. Severe injury or major surgery can affect male fertility, as can certain diseases or conditions, such as diabetes, thyroid disease, HIV/AIDS, Cushing's disease, anemia, heart attack, and liver or kidney failure. In addition, radiation and chemotherapy treatment for cancer can impair sperm production. The closer radiation treatment is to the testicles, the higher the risk of infertility. Removal of testicles because of cancer also may affect male fertility.

Like women, a man's general health and lifestyle may affect fertility, though in different ways. Alcohol, drugs, and tobacco use are associated with reduced fertility. Alcohol can reduce testosterone levels and reduce the quality and quantity of sperm. Anabolic steroids, which are taken to stimulate muscle strength and growth, can cause the testicles to shrink and sperm production to decrease. Marijuana is thought to decrease sperm density and motility and increase sperm abnormalities. Cocaine and opiates contribute to erectile dysfunction, and amphetamines can decrease sex drive. Smoking may increase infertility and erectile dysfunction, as well as affect the form of sperm and speed at which they move.

Another common factor that affects men and women is an increased body mass. We will discuss weight, BMI, and weight distribution and its effects on fertility in Chapter 2. In addition, weight may interfere with certain hormones needed to produce sperm.

Your sperm count may be affected if you experience excessive or prolonged emotional stress. A problem with fertility itself can sometimes become long term and discouraging, producing more stress. Infertility can affect social relationships and sexual functioning.

Dietary deficiencies may also play a role. Many antioxidant nutrients (discussed in Chapter 4) promote proper sperm form and function. Nutrients affecting the quality and quantity of sperm include vitamin C, vitamin E, selenium, zinc, folate, vitamin B_{12}, plus omega-3 fatty acids and specific amino acids. Deficiencies in these nutrients may contribute to infertility. Be sure to check out Chapter 5, where we focus specifically on how men can increase their vitality through diet.

Two things that men should also watch out for include pesticides and other chemicals and testicular exposure to overheating. Herbicides and insecticides used in agriculture not grown organically may have estrogen-like activity and cause female-hormonelike effects in the male body, reducing sperm production. Exposure to such chemicals also may contribute to testicular cancer. Men exposed to hydrocarbons, such as ethylbenzene, benzene, toluene, xylene, and aromatic solvents used in paint, varnishes, glues, metal degreasers, and other products, may be at risk of infertility. Men with high exposure to lead also may be more at risk.

Frequent use of saunas, hot tubs, or hot baths can elevate a man's core body temperature, which may impair sperm production and lower the sperm count. Bicycling more than thirty minutes at a time also raises scrotal temperature and negatively affects sperm production.

Ovulation Issues: How to Chart Your Fertility Pattern

Conception requires an intricate series of events, so many factors may be responsible for a delay in starting your family. Each month, the pituitary gland in a woman's brain sends a signal to her ovaries to prepare an egg for ovulation. The pituitary produces two hormones that are involved in stimulating the ovaries to bring an egg to ovulation: the *follicle-stimulating hormone* (*FSH*) and *luteinizing hormone* (*LH*). A surge in LH relays a message to the ovarian follicle to release its egg (ovulate). A woman is most fertile at the time of ovulation—around day fourteen of her menstrual cycle—although the exact time of ovulation varies among women because of different lengths of menstrual cycles.

After the egg is released into the follicle, it is then captured by a fallopian tube and is viable for about twenty-four hours, with its best time for fertilization within the first twelve hours following ovulation. For pregnancy to occur, a sperm must unite with the egg in the fallopian tube within this time frame. Sperm are capable of fertilizing the egg for up to seventy-two hours and must be present in the fallopian tube at the same time as the egg for conception to occur. If fertilized, the egg moves into the uterus two to four days later where it attaches to the uterine lining and begins a nine-month process of growth.

A woman being aware of her menstrual cycle and the changes in her body that happen during this time can be key to helping plan or avoid pregnancy. During the menstrual cycle (a total average of twenty-eight days), there are two parts: before ovulation and after ovulation.

* **Day 1** starts with the first day of a woman's period.
* **Usually by day 7**, a woman's eggs start to prepare to be fertilized by sperm.
* **Between days 7 and 11**, the lining of the uterus (womb) starts to thicken, waiting for a fertilized egg to implant there.
* **Around day 14** (in a twenty-eight-day cycle), hormones cause the egg that is most ripe to be released, a process called ovulation. The egg travels down the fallopian tube toward the uterus. If a sperm unites with the egg here, the egg will attach to the lining of the uterus, and pregnancy occurs. If the egg is not fertilized, it will break apart.

✤ **Around day 25** when hormone levels drop, the egg will be shed from the body with the lining of the uterus as a menstrual period.

The first part of the menstrual cycle is different in every woman and can even be different from month to month in the same woman, varying from thirteen to twenty days long. This is the most important part of the cycle to learn about, because this is when ovulation and pregnancy can occur. After ovulation, every woman (unless she has a health problem that affects her periods) will have a period within fourteen to sixteen days.

If a woman is aware of when she is most fertile, she can try to plan or prevent a pregnancy. There are three ways that a woman can keep track of this time each month: basal body temperature, calendar method, and cervical mucus method (also known as the ovulation method).

Basal Body Temperature Method

This method involves a woman taking her *basal body temperature* (the body's temperature when at rest) every morning before she gets out of bed and recording it on a chart. A woman usually begins to know her own fertility pattern and can see the changes from month to month.

During the menstrual cycle, her body temperature remains at a somewhat steady, lower level and begins to slightly rise with ovulation. The rise can be a sudden jump or a gradual climb over a few days. The rise in temperature can't predict exactly when the egg is released, but her temperature rises between 0.4 to 0.8 degree Fahrenheit on the day of ovulation. She is most fertile and most likely to get pregnant during the two to three days just before her temperature hits the highest point (ovulation) and for about twelve to twenty-four hours after ovulation. A man's sperm can live for up to three days in her body and is able to fertilize an egg during that time. So, if a woman has unprotected sex several days before ovulation, there is a chance of becoming pregnant. Once her temperature spikes and stays at a higher level for about three days, she can be sure that ovulation has occurred. Her temperature will remain at the higher level until her period starts.

Basal body temperature differs slightly from woman to woman, but anywhere from 96 to 98 degrees orally is normal before ovulation, and anywhere from 97 to 99 degrees orally after ovulation. So, any charted changes are very small and are in 1/10 degree. An oral basal body temperature thermometer or an easy-to-read thermometer, which has the degrees marked in these small fractions, can be purchased at a drugstore. If you can't find it easily, ask the pharmacist to help you.

Calendar Method

This method involves keeping a written record of each menstrual cycle on a regular calendar. The first day of a woman's period is day 1, which can be circled on the calendar. This should be continued for eight to twelve months so she can know how many days are in her cycle. The length of her cycle can vary from month to month, so she should write down the total number of days it lasts each time in a list.

To find out the first day when a woman is most fertile, check the list and find the cycle with the fewest days. Then subtract eighteen from that number. Take this new number and count ahead that many days on the calendar. Draw an X through this date. The X marks the first day a woman is likely to be fertile.

To find out the last day when a woman is fertile, subtract eleven days from the longest cycle and draw an X through this date. This method always should be used with other fertility awareness methods, especially if the cycles are not always the same lengths.

Cervical Mucus Method (Ovulation Method)

This method involves being aware of the changes in the cervical mucus throughout the month. The hormones that control the menstrual cycle also cause changes in the consistency and amount of mucus that occurs just before and during ovulation. Right after a period, a woman usually has a few days when there is no mucus present or "dry days." As the egg starts to mature, mucus increases in the vagina, appears at the vaginal opening, and is usually white or yellow and cloudy and sticky. The greatest amount of mucus appears just before ovulation, during the "wet days," when it becomes clear and slippery, like raw egg whites. Sometimes it can be stretched apart, and this is when she is most fertile.

About four days after the wet days begin, the mucus changes again. There is now much less and it becomes sticky and cloudy. She might have a few more dry days before her period returns. Changes in mucus can be described on a calendar. Label the days, "sticky," "dry," or "wet." A woman is most fertile at the first sign of wetness after her period but may be also a day or two before wetness begins.

This method is less reliable for women whose mucus pattern is changed because of breast-feeding, use of oral contraceptives or feminine hygiene products, having vaginitis, sexually transmitted diseases (STDs), or surgery on the cervix.

To most accurately track fertility, it is best to use a combination of all three methods, which is called the *symptothermal method.*

Tests for Infertility

Don't wait to see the doctor if you suspect a fertility problem, especially if you are over thirty-five. A medical evaluation may determine the reasons for a couple's infertility. Typically, the process begins with physical exams and medical and sexual histories of both partners. If the problem is not obvious, like improperly timed intercourse or absence of ovulation (*anovulation*), additional tests may be needed.

For men, doctors will run a battery of tests, usually beginning with evaluation of semen to look at the number, shape, and movement of his sperm. Other kinds of tests, including hormone tests, are also done.

For a woman, the first step in uncovering a fertility problem is to test to find out if she is ovulating each month. There are several ways to do this. For example, she can keep track of changes in her morning body temperature and in the texture of her cervical mucus. Another tool is a home ovulation test kit, which can be bought at drug or grocery stores. You may also want to use an online ovulation calculator provided by the government (visit 4woman.gov/pregnancy/ovulation1.cfm) to gauge your personal ovulation peak, based on your cycle. This calculator will then give you a good idea of when you are ovulating.

Tests for ovulation can also be done in the doctor's office, using blood tests for hormone levels or ultrasound tests of the ovaries. Remember, 25 percent of infertility is related to ovulation, which can be assisted with lifestyle factors, such as diet and achievement of a healthy weight, as well as prescription drugs. Some common hormone level tests to determine ovulation include:

* Follicle-stimulating hormone (FSH)
* Luteinizing hormone (LH)
* Estrogen
* Testosterone
* Progesterone

If the woman is ovulating, more tests will need to be done. Some common female tests include:

✢ **Hysterosalpingogram.** An x-ray of the fallopian tubes and uterus after they are injected with dye. It shows if the tubes are open and shows the shape of the uterus.

✢ **Laparoscopy.** An exam of the tubes and other female organs for disease. An instrument called a laparoscope is used to see inside the abdomen.

Treating Infertility

Depending on the test results, different treatments can be suggested. Approximately 85 to 90 percent of infertility cases are treated with drugs or surgery. A number of fertility drugs may be used for women with ovulation problems. It is important to talk with your health-care provider about the drug to be used and make sure you understand the drug's benefits and side effects. Depending on the type of fertility drug and the dosage of the drug used, multiple births (such as twins) can occur in some women.

If needed, surgery can be done to repair damage to a woman's ovaries, fallopian tubes, or uterus. A man with an infertility problems may also have surgical options.

Fertility Medications

Fertility drugs are the primary treatment for women who are infertile because of ovulation disorders. By inducing ovulation, they exert action designed to work like natural FSH and LH. Some of the commonly used fertility drugs are:

✢ **Clomiphene citrate** (Clomid, Serophene) stimulates ovulation in women who have PCOS or other ovulatory disorders. This drug causes the pituitary gland to release more FSH and LH, stimulating the growth of an ovarian follicle containing an egg. It is taken orally.

✤ **Human menopausal gonadotropin, or hMG** (Repronex, Pergonal), directly stimulates the ovaries for women who don't menstruate because of failure of the pituitary gland to fulfill its role in inducing ovulation. This drug is injected.

✤ **Follicle-stimulating hormone (FSH)** (Gonal-F, Follistim, Bravelle) stimulates the ovaries to mature egg follicles. FSH is essentially hMG (a gonadotropin) without the LH.

✤ **Human chorionic gonadotropin, or hCG** (Ovidrel, Pregnyl), stimulates the follicle to release its egg (ovulate) and is used in combination with clomiphene, hMG, and FSH.

✤ **Gonadotropin-releasing hormone (Gn-RH) analogs** is a treatment prescribed for women with irregular ovulatory cycles or who ovulate prematurely during hMG treatment. Delivering constant gonadotropin-releasing hormone to the pituitary gland alters hormone production, so that a physician can induce follicle growth with FSH.

✤ **Bromocriptine** is a medication for women with elevated levels of prolactin, which cause irregular ovulation cycles. By reducing prolactin, ovulation can become more regular and increase the chances of pregnancy.

Assisted Reproductive Technology (ART)

Assisted reproductive technology (ART) involves both the woman's eggs and the man's sperm, and success rates vary and depend on many factors. ART can be rather expensive and time-consuming but has made conception a possibility for many couples.

In vitro fertilization (IVF) is used for a variety of fertility problems. This procedure was made famous with the 1978 birth of Louise Brown, the world's first "test tube baby." A drug is used to stimulate the ovaries to produce multiple eggs, which upon maturation are combined with sperm outside the uterus for fertilization. After about forty hours, the eggs are examined to see if they have become fertilized by the sperm and are dividing into cells. These fertilized eggs (*embryos*) are then placed in the woman's uterus, thus bypassing the fallopian tubes.

Gamete intrafallopian transfer (*GIFT*) is similar to IVF but used when the woman has at least one normal fallopian tube. Three to five eggs are placed in the fallopian tube, along with the sperm, for fertilization to occur inside the woman's body.

Zygote intrafallopian transfer (*ZIFT*), also called *tubal embryo transfer*, combines IVF and GIFT. The eggs taken from the woman's ovaries are fertilized in the lab and then placed in the fallopian tubes rather than the uterus.

How You Can Eat to Boost Fertility

Although physical defects affecting fertility (such as blocked fallopian tubes) cannot be assisted by diet, research is showing that when ovulation—an endocrine issue—is a culprit, as it is in 25 percent of infertility cases, lifestyle can play a role in achieving pregnancy. Because the endocrine system—the intricate superhighway of hormones in the body—affects reproduction, and because what we eat plays a big role in the function of our endocrine system, science is emerging that shows *we can eat to boost fertility*. In the next chapter, we'll discuss some of the barriers to fertility and how they are affected by diet.

Barriers to Conception: PCOS, Insulin Resistance, and Other Hormonal Factors

THE ENDOCRINE SYSTEM is made up of glands that produce and secrete hormones. The major glands of the endocrine system are the *hypothalamus, pituitary, thyroid, parathyroids, adrenals, pineal,* and the *reproductive organs* (ovaries and testes). The pancreas is also a part of this system and produces insulin, which has many effects on your weight, reproductive capabilities, and ability to have a successful pregnancy. The hormones secreted from the endocrine system regulate the body's growth and metabolism, as well as sexual development and reproductive capabilities.

Like a pinball machine, hormones are released into the bloodstream and along the way affect many other hormones or organs throughout the body, causing a chain of events. The purpose of hormones is to send messages to coordinate functions to different parts of the body. One wrong turn in the proverbial pinball machine of our endocrine system can cause a number of health problems, many of which are, not surprisingly, interrelated. For example, thyroid dysfunction (both an underactive thyroid and an overactive thyroid) can cause irregular menstrual cycles, affect a woman's ability to conceive, and contribute to the risk of miscarriage. Simple blood tests can be obtained to determine how normally the thyroid is functioning.

Problems with the endocrine system can impair fertility, but the good news is that once a problem is discovered, it may be managed to restore fertility and decrease the risk of associated pregnancy complications. In this chapter we'll focus on the interrelated aspects of the endocrine system, how it affects your fertility, and the dietary measures that may boost your fertility. We'll also discuss other barriers to conception, including polycystic ovary syndrome (PCOS), inflammation, insulin resistance (a condition that makes your body less sensitive to the effects of insulin), and endometriosis, which scientists believe are also diet related.

How Weight and Body Mass Index Affect Infertility

The American Society for Reproductive Medicine says that a weight loss of 5 to 10 percent can dramatically improve ovulation and pregnancy rates, as well as reduce the risk for diabetes, heart disease, and high blood pressure. Being overweight or obese can have serious consequences for the reproductive system and pregnancy including:

+ Irregular or infrequent menstrual cycles
+ Lack of ovulation (anovulation)
+ Decreased success with fertility treatment
+ Increased risk of miscarriage
+ Increased risk of high blood pressure
+ Increased risk of diabetes in pregnancy

❖ Increased risk of birth defects
❖ Increased risk of high birth-weight infant
❖ Increased risk of Cesarean section

So, how does being overweight affect your fertility? *Adipocytes*, or fat cells, shoot out inflammatory factors called *cytokines*. Like wounding bullets, these cytokines (including tumor necrosis factor, interleukin, and C-reactive protein [CRP]) get in the way of normal bodily functions and have negative effects on hormones. When more fat cells are present, cytokines are released, resulting in a state of inflammation. Research has revealed that inflammation is related to a number of other conditions such as insulin resistance, type 2 diabetes, cardiovascular disease, and metabolic syndrome. Let's take a look at how your weight affects the endocrine system, ovulation, and your pregnancy.

Weight Distribution, Ovulation, and Infertility

Of special importance to your fertility appears to be the distribution of weight. Abdominal obesity, long known to contribute to insulin resistance and diabetes, is also being examined for its role in infertility as well as endometrial cancer and breast cancer.

Although the mechanisms are still not completely understood, scientists know that being overweight or obese increases insulin levels and *androgens* (male hormones including testosterone), as well as those inflammatory compounds produced by fat cells we discussed. The result is lack of ovulation and reduced fertility. But the good news is that research shows weight loss through diet and exercise can help get you back on track, stabilize insulin levels, and boost your fertility.

How Exercise Can Improve Ovulation

In 2002, the Nurses' Health Study II conducted by Harvard estimated that 25 percent of ovulatory infertility is related to being overweight. The study examined physical activity and body fat as risk factors for infertility due to problems with ovulation. The study compared 830 cases of ovulatory infertility and 26,125 pregnancies. The study showed that an increase in vigorous activity decreased the risk of ovulatory infertility. In fact, thirty minutes per week of vigorous activity was found to be associated with a 7 percent reduction in infertility relating to ovulatory issues.

Polycystic Ovary Syndrome (PCOS) and Infertility

PCOS is a common hormone imbalance that is best known for causing infertility and estimated to affect 5 to 10 percent of women of reproductive age.

A growing collection of research shows that elevated insulin levels contribute to increased androgen production by a woman's ovaries and have a causative role in PCOS. Studies also indicate that women whose sisters have PCOS are more likely to develop the condition, and that PCOS increases the risk of certain cancers, diabetes, and heart disease.

Affecting the Reproductive System

Women with PCOS often have the following reproductive problems that impede fertility:

✢ **Amenorrhea (no menstrual period), infrequent menses, and/or oligomenorrhea (infrequent ovulation leading to irregular bleeding).** These menstrual cycles are usually greater than six weeks in length, with eight or fewer periods in a year. Irregular bleeding may include lengthy bleeding episodes, scant or heavy periods, or frequent spotting.

✤ **Hyperandrogenism.** Women with PCOS have increased serum levels of male hormones, specifically, testosterone, androstenedione, and dehydroepiandrosterone sulfate (DHEAS).

✤ **Cystic or enlarged ovaries.** Typical PCOS ovaries have a "string of pearls" appearance with many cysts (fluid-filled sacs); women with PCOS have ovaries that are usually 1½ to 3 times larger than normal.

✤ **Oligo or anovulation (infrequent or absent ovulation).** The follicles produced by women with PCOS often do not mature and release as needed for ovulation. With PCOS, infertility (the inability to get pregnant within six to twelve months of unprotected intercourse, depending on age) is usually due to ovulatory dysfunction.

A woman's ovaries have follicles, which are tiny, fluid-filled sacs that hold the eggs. When an egg is mature, the follicle breaks open to release the egg so it can travel to the uterus for fertilization. In women with PCOS, immature follicles bunch together to form large cysts or lumps. The eggs mature within the bunched follicles, but the follicles don't break open to release them. Thus, because the eggs are not released, most women with PCOS have trouble getting pregnant.

Additional Key Symptoms

Although best known for causing infertility, women with PCOS may also have other health problems, such as abnormally high levels of insulin, obesity, high blood pressure, and heart disease. Most of these women will also gain weight and notice an increase in their hair growth. Let's take a look at some of the other health symptoms.

✤ **Obesity or weight gain.** Women with PCOS will have what is called an apple figure where excess weight is concentrated heavily in the abdomen, similar to the way men often gain weight, with comparatively narrower arms and legs. Most, but not all, women with PCOS are overweight.

❖ **Chronic pelvic pain.** Enlarged ovaries may lead to pelvic pressure and pain; it is considered chronic when it has continued for more than six months.

❖ **Insulin resistance, hyperinsulinemia, and diabetes.** Insulin resistance is an inability for the body to use insulin efficiently and is usually accompanied by compensatory hyperinsulinemia—an overproduction of insulin.

❖ **Dyslipidemia (lipid abnormalities) and hypertension.** Some women with PCOS have elevated LDL and reduced HDL cholesterol levels, as well as high triglycerides. Some also have high blood pressure readings over 140/90.

❖ **Excess hair and male-pattern baldness or thinning hair.** Excess hair growth (*hirsutism*) can appear on the face, chest, abdomen, thumbs, or toes. In addition, women with PCOS may experience balding (*alopecia*)—most commonly on the top of the head rather than at the temples.

❖ **Skin problems.** Overproduction of androgens stimulates oil production on the skin as well as acne. *Seborrhea* causes dandruff —flaking skin on the scalp caused by excess oil. Women with PCOS may also encounter dark patches of skin, tan to dark brown or black (*acanthosis nigricans*)—typically on the back of the neck but also in skin creases under arms, breasts, and between thighs, and occasionally on the hands, elbows, and knees. The darkened skin is usually velvety or rough to the touch. Tiny flaps or skin tags (*acrochordons*) can also appear that usually cause no symptoms unless irritated by rubbing.

Tests for PCOS

The blood work that should be done in diagnosing or ruling out PCOS is the same as a basic fertility workup. However, there are a couple of additional tests for insulin resistance that should be added, as well as some cholesterol screening to evaluate general health status because of the future risks associated with PCOS. A screening may include:

- ❖ Fasting comprehensive biochemical and lipid panel
- ❖ Two-hour glucose tolerance test (GTT) with insulin levels (also called IGTT)
- ❖ LH:FSH ratio
- ❖ Total testosterone
- ❖ DHEAS
- ❖ SHBG
- ❖ Androstenedione
- ❖ Prolactin
- ❖ Thyroid stimulating hormone (TSH)

Insulin Resistance: Linked with PCOS, Inflammation, and Hormones

It is estimated that 20 to 40 percent of women with PCOS have impaired insulin function—a number seven times higher than women without the condition. As we discussed earlier in the chapter, hormones produce a cascade of events in the body. As the body produces more insulin, it signals an increase in androgens. The androgens, being male hormones, reduce the maturation of follicles, inhibit ovulation, and produce more cysts. A number of inflammatory factors have an effect on insulin resistance, which is associated with PCOS. In this section we'll take a look at those compounds, their relationship to PCOS, and later reveal the research on how diet can help to break the barriers to conception.

C-reactive protein (*CRP*) is one of the inflammatory factors in the body associated with insulin resistance. A 2004 study published in the journal *Hormone Research* evaluated women with PCOS and found significantly higher levels of this dangerous inflammatory factor in their blood along with the presence of insulin resistance.

Adiponectin, a peptide that improves insulin sensitivity, has anti-inflammatory action and is associated with a lower risk of heart disease and diabetes. A 2005 study published in *Obstetrical and Gynecological Survey* found that low levels of adiponectin might contribute to or worsen the development of insulin resistance and play a role in PCOS. Harvard doctors looked at the association between diet and adiponectin and they found that a carbohydrate-rich diet with a high glycemic load is associated with lower levels of this insulin-sensitizing compound in people without heart disease. We'll discuss the glycemic load in Chapter 3 and provide you with recipes and meal plans at the end of the book that can help to balance your blood sugar.

Leptin, a hormone decoded from the obesity gene, has also been found to have an effect on fertility. Secreted exclusively from fat (or adipose) tissue, this hormone acts on the central nervous system to suppress food intake and increase energy consumption. Studies show that animals lacking leptin develop obesity and become infertile. Recent studies show that zinc—a mineral long known for its role in reproduction—helps to boost leptin levels.

Ghrelin is a hormone involved in appetite regulation and PCOS. A recent study found that women without PCOS had 70 percent higher levels of ghrelin than women with PCOS. The participants with PCOS were less satiated and hungrier after a meal than those without PCOS, suggesting appetite regulation is also involved with PCOS.

Endometriosis and Fertility

Endometriosis is a painful, chronic disease that affects 5½ million women in the United States and millions more worldwide. Endometriosis occurs when tissues inside the uterus grow outside the uterus. These tissues can deposit themselves in the organs in the abdominal areas and in other places they're not supposed to grow. The word *endometriosis* comes from the word *endometrium* —*endo* meaning "inside," and *metrium* meaning "mother." Health-care providers call the tissue that lines the inside of the uterus (where a mother carries her baby) the endometrium. They may also call areas of endometriosis by different names, such as *implants, lesions,* or *nodules.*

Examining Symptoms and Causes

One of the most common symptoms of endometriosis is pain, mostly in the abdomen, lower back, and pelvic areas. The amount of pain a woman feels is not linked to how much endometriosis she has. Some women have no pain even though their endometriosis is extensive, meaning that the affected areas are large or that there is scarring. On the other hand, some women have severe pain even though they have only a few small areas of endometriosis.

General symptoms of endometriosis can include (but are not limited to):

* Extremely painful (or disabling) menstrual cramps (pain may get worse over time)
* Chronic pelvic pain (includes lower back pain and pelvic pain)
* Pain during or after sex
* Intestinal pain
* Painful bowel movements or painful urination during menstrual periods
* Heavy menstrual periods
* Premenstrual spotting or bleeding between periods
* Infertility

In addition, women who are diagnosed with endometriosis may have gastrointestinal symptoms that resemble a bowel disorder, as well as fatigue.

Endometriosis may result from something called "retrograde menstrual flow," in which some of the tissue that a woman sheds during her period flows into her pelvis. While most women who get their periods have some retrograde menstrual flow, not all of these women have endometriosis. Researchers are trying to uncover what other factors might cause the tissue to grow in some women but not in others.

Another theory about the cause of endometriosis involves genes. This disease could be inherited or it could result from genetic errors, making some women more likely than others to develop the condition. If researchers can find a specific gene or genes related to endometriosis in some women, genetic testing might allow health-care providers to detect endometriosis much earlier, or even prevent it from happening at all.

Researchers are exploring other possible causes, as well. Estrogen, a hormone involved in the female reproductive cycle, appears to promote the growth of endometriosis. Therefore, some research is looking into endometriosis as a disease of the endocrine system. Or, it may be that a woman's immune system does not remove the menstrual fluid in the pelvic cavity properly; or the chemicals made by areas of endometriosis may irritate or promote growth of more areas. As a result, some researchers are studying the role of the immune system in either stimulating or reacting to endometriosis.

Other research focuses on determining whether environmental agents, such as exposure to man-made chemicals, cause endometriosis. Understanding what, if any, factors influence the course of the disease is being sought.

Tests for Endometriosis

Currently, health-care providers use a number of tests for endometriosis. Sometimes, they will use imaging tests to produce a "picture" of the inside of the body, which allows them to locate larger endometriosis areas, such as nodules or cysts. The two most common imaging tests are *ultrasound*, a machine that uses sound waves to make the picture, and *magnetic resonance imaging (MRI)*, a machine that uses magnets and radio waves to make the picture.

The only way to know for sure that a woman has the condition is by having surgery. The most common type of surgery is called *laparoscopy*. After making a small cut in the abdomen through the belly button, the surgeon uses a small viewing instrument with a light, called a *laparoscope*, to look at the reproductive organs, intestines, and other surfaces to see if there is any endometriosis. He or she can make a diagnosis based on the characteristic appearance of endometriosis. This diagnosis can then be confirmed by doing a biopsy, which involves taking a small tissue sample and studying it under a microscope.

The health-care provider will only do a laparoscopy after learning the full medical history and giving a complete physical and pelvic exam. This information, in addition to the results of an ultrasound or MRI, will help the patient and her health-care provider make more informed decisions about treatment.

How Inflammation and Diet Can Affect Endometriosis

As we found with PCOS, endometriosis is also affected by inflammation. A 2004 Yale study found that fluid collected from women with endometriosis had higher levels of immune cells, called *macrophages*, and their accompanying secreted products including cytokines, growth factors, and factors that encourage new blood vessel formation (angiogenesis). Because reproductive organs are bathed in these fluids, the inflammatory factors affect reproductive capability in women with endometriosis.

Two studies published in *Human Reproduction* (Oxford, England) examined different aspects of endometriosis. One evaluated levels of C-reactive protein (CRP) for diagnosing endo-

metriosis and found higher levels of CRP in women with endometriosis than in those without the disease. The other recent
study published evaluated 504 women with endometriosis. The
participants were asked about their diet in the previous year,
including weekly portions of selected items, specific nutrients
including carotenoids and retinoids, as well as alcohol and coffee. Compared with the women with the lowest intake, the risk
of endometriosis was significantly lower for those women eating
the most green vegetables and fresh fruit (sources of carotenoids
and retinoids). Beef and other red meat, as well as ham, were
associated with an increased risk of endometriosis.

Reducing Inflammation Through Diet

Thus far in the chapter, we've discussed the relationship between
inflammation and two pregnancy barriers: PCOS and endometriosis. Let's take a look at the research on reducing inflammation through diet.

In a study, 732 healthy women from the Nurses' Health
Study were evaluated using a food-frequency questionnaire—a
tool that analyzes what foods they ate and how often they ate
them. The study compared women consuming a "prudent" pattern diet—higher intakes of fruit, vegetables, legumes, fish, poultry, and whole grains—with those consuming a Western pattern
diet—characterized by higher intakes of red and processed meats,
sweets, desserts, french fries, and refined grains. The prudent pattern was associated with lower levels of CRP, whereas the Western pattern showed a positive relation with CRP (and other
markers of inflammation). Partly because of their diverse mix of
phytonutrients, veggie vigilantes, and fruits, too; the prudent pattern diet helped to reduce those inflammatory factors that
increase the risk for insulin resistance, diabetes, and heart disease.

A recent study conducted at the Jean Mayer U.S. Department of Agriculture, Human Nutrition Research Center on Aging at Tufts examined the relationship between CRP, another inflammatory factor called homocysteine, and the intake of fruits and vegetables. The study found that frequent consumption of fruits and vegetables is associated with lower concentrations of both CRP and homocysteine.

One group of phytonutrients (plant nutrients) in particular, the flavonoids, has been studied for their anti-inflammatory action. We'll learn about the diverse flavonoids in foods that can help balance your blood sugar in Chapter 4.

Similarly, the National Health and Nutrition Examination Survey (NHANES) found that fiber intake was inversely associated with CRP levels. We have many recipes that are loaded with fiber that we'll point out to you in Chapter 10. The Health Eating Index (HEI)—a measure of diet quality according to the Dietary Guidelines for Americans—was examined for its effect on CRP. Among the components measured, researchers concluded that grain consumption may reduce inflammation, as whole-grain consumption was inversely associated with CRP levels.

Studies on metabolism have shown that a high intake of rapidly digested and absorbed carbohydrates can lead to insulin resistance. These quickly digested carbohydrates—ranking high on a scale called the *glycemic index*—rapidly deliver sugar to the bloodstream, causing insulin levels to spike. In the next chapter, we discuss the glycemic index, which was created to quantify and rank the body's response to different carbohydrate-containing foods. In later chapters, we'll talk about the nutrients and foods to arm yourself with for a fertility-boosting arsenal.

Fats, Carbs, and Your Fertility

ACCORDING TO THE National Vital Statistics Reports, infertility is on the rise. Just as Americans are having a harder time conceiving, the rates of diabetes and heart disease are also continuing to climb. Is there a link? Sectors of the scientific community think so, and they believe the answer lies in insulin resistance spurred by the wrong kinds of fats and carbs in the diet.

Over the past few decades, mixed messages on fats and carbohydrates have led many Americans down a road of degenerating health. First, we hear that fat is bad, and carbohydrates (or carbs) are good. Then, we are fed the notion that severely limiting carbs—and all the wonderfully nutritious foods they are found in—will help us lose weight. A healthy weight is a key factor in preventing disease. Unfortunately, an astounding two-thirds of Americans are overweight and infertility now affects 6.1 million Americans (or 10 percent of the reproductive age population). The truth of the matter and common denominator among fats and carbs is this: *there are healthy ones and there are unhealthy ones.*

The glycemic index (GI), a new system for classifying carbs, gives us greater insight to the all-carbs-are-bad myth and helps us separate the wheat from the chaff (no pun intended). By measuring how fast and how high blood sugar rises after consuming a carb-rich food, we better understand the impact foods have on insulin and the health issues surrounding insulin, including fertility.

Although such a system does not exist for fats, numerous studies have proven the "friends" and "foes" of the fat world. Fats have the ability to increase or decrease insulin, alter the number of ovarian follicles, affect ovulation rate, and impact progesterone production by the corpus luteum (the area in the ovary where the egg is released at ovulation). Dietary fats (along with other factors, including excess calories and unhealthy carbohydrates) also play a role in the development of gestational diabetes, affecting the quality of mother's milk and the intelligence of the unborn child. Research shows the same fats that protect a woman's heart and keep her insulin levels in check also help to boost fertility. We'll discuss specific dietary fats affecting male fertility in Chapter 5.

When a woman eliminates healthy carbs and healthy fats, she also forgoes the critical nutrients that help to balance blood sugar and support pregnancy and the health of her baby. Afraid of fat so she skips the olive oil, nuts, and avocados? She's missing out on minerals such as magnesium, good fats, plus antioxidants. Under the impression that all carbs are bad? There goes the fiber and phytoestrogens that work together to keep blood sugar on an even keel.

Healing Gourmet makes it easy to follow the principles discovered by modern science to benefit fertility. You will notice that we reference a number of large epidemiological studies throughout. In this chapter, we will point out the good guys and bad guys of the fat and carb world and how they relate to insulin resistance and ovulatory infertility.

How Unhealthy Fats Can Lead to Infertility

Structurally, fats are simple molecules built around a series of carbon atoms (C) linked to each other in a chain. Dietary fats are composed of long chains containing twelve to twenty-two carbons. A small change in the structure of a dietary fat can make a big impact on overall health. First, let's take a look at the fat foes and their effects on fertility.

The Fat Foe: Saturated Fat

Saturated fats are mainly animal fats. They are found in meat, whole milk dairy products (such as cheese, milk, and ice cream), poultry skin, and egg yolks. Some plant foods are also high in saturated fats, including coconut and coconut oil, palm oil, and palm kernel oil. With saturated fatty acids, each of the interior carbon atoms is bonded to two hydrogen atoms as well as two other carbons. All of the bonds available for hydrogen are filled or "saturated" with hydrogen, hence the name.

Saturated fat in the diet stifles the function of the insulin-secreting cells of the pancreas (beta cells), reducing sensitivity to insulin. As we consume saturated fats, they are stored in cells as triglycerides, causing damage to those cells. As these compounds increase in our insulin-secreting cells, the damage accumulates and causes these important cells to die, worsening insulin resistance and PCOS.

The recent study published in *Human Reproduction* (that we mentioned in Chapter 2) also points to saturated fats as a culprit for infertility relating to endometriosis. The researchers believe that saturated fats increase estrogens and also affect prostaglandin function and the functioning of the ovaries. This study particularly examined the saturated fat in beef, other red meats, and ham.

Not by coincidence, the Health Professionals Follow-Up Study found a relationship between dietary fat and meat intake to the risk of type 2 diabetes. The study followed 42,504 male participants for twelve years and found total and saturated fat intakes were associated with a higher risk of type 2 diabetes. The study also showed that frequently eating processed meats—such as lunch meat, hot dogs, or bacon—may increase the risk for type 2 diabetes.

Similarly, the Women's Health Study examined the relationship between red-meat consumption and risk of type 2 diabetes. Over an eight-year, eight-month period, 37,309 female participants—age forty-five or older who were free of disease (including cancer, heart disease, and type 2 diabetes)—were given food-frequency questionnaires (a survey of the types and amounts of foods eaten). The study showed that eating red and processed meats significantly increased the risk for type 2 diabetes, emphasizing a higher risk for those who frequently ate processed meat, including bacon and hot dogs. (We'll discuss the dangers of processed meats and pregnancy more in Chapter 7.)

Another study (published in *Human Reproduction*) evaluated the fat composition of failed eggs in women undergoing in vitro fertilization (IVF). A total of 150 unfertilized oocytes (eggs before maturation) were analyzed. When researchers looked at the composition of fats in the embryos, they discovered the majority of the fats in those eggs were saturated fats (stearic and palmitic). In the study, the fatty acids in the lowest concentrations were the healthy fats—polyunsaturated and monounsaturated fats.

 Healing Tip

By limiting or avoiding red meat, processed meat, and full-fat dairy, you can minimize your exposure to the beta-cell bully, saturated fat. Opt instead for plant-based fats, fish, low-fat dairy, and lean poultry—preferably organic or free range. We'll talk further about the benefits of organic and free-range foods for pregnancy more in Chapter 7.

The Foe: Trans Fat

Trans fatty acids are fats produced through a process called *hydrogenation*, which adds hydrogen to the fat molecule. Hydrogenation became popular because this type of oil doesn't spoil or become rancid as easily as regular oil and therefore has a longer shelf life. The more hydrogenated an oil is, the harder it will be at room temperature. For example, a spreadable tub of margarine is less hydrogenated and so has fewer trans fats than a stick of margarine. Most of the trans fats in the American diet are found in commercially prepared baked goods, margarines, snack foods, and processed foods, as well as commercially prepared fried foods—such as french fries and onion rings.

A report from the Institute of Medicine concluded that there is no safe level of trans fats in the diet. This prompted the FDA to require that all Nutrition Facts food labels include trans fats by January 1, 2006. Check food labels for hydrogenated oils; the higher on the list they appear, the more trans fats there are in the product. We talk more about understanding the labeling on foods in Chapter 8.

Irrefutably, eating foods containing trans fats increases the risk for heart disease because of the action of these villainous fats on cholesterol and inflammation. They are also being examined for their negative impact on blood sugar, insulin, and inflammation. The Nurses' Healthy Study evaluated 823 women for markers of inflammation and found that eating trans fat–containing foods increases C-reactive protein (CRP), which, as we discussed in Chapter 2, is associated with PCOS and endometriosis. CRP is most well known for its negative contribution to heart disease and diabetes.

The FDA based these trans fats guidelines on recent studies that indicate that consumption of trans fatty acids contributes to increased LDL cholesterol levels, which increase the risk of coronary heart disease. Recent information from the American Heart Association indicates that heart disease causes about 500,000 deaths annually and is the number-one cause of death in the United States. Thus, the FDA is proposing to provide for information on trans fatty acids in nutrition labeling and nutrient content and health claims in response to its importance to public health.

Because women with PCOS have an increased risk of heart disease and diabetes, avoiding these stealthy fats can not only help boost fertility but also evade major health consequences. Table 3.1 illustrates the amounts of trans fats in common foods.

 Healing Tip

To reduce the inflammatory factors associated with chronic diseases, root out trans fat by looking for "partially hydrogenated oils" or "vegetable shortening" on food labels. Look in your local grocery store for trans fat–free shortenings and baked goods.

Healthy Fats to Boost Fertility

Let's take a look at the health-promoting fats that benefit insulin function and help reduce inflammatory processes involved with PCOS, endometriosis, pregnancy, miscarriage, and other chronic diseases.

The Friend: Monounsaturated Fats (MUFAs)

Monounsaturated fats (MUFAs) are derived from vegetable sources including olives, nuts, and avocados. The double bond in these fats allows the monounsaturated fatty acid chain to be a bit

TABLE 3.1 Trans Fatty Acids in One Serving of Selected Foods	
Food	Trans Fatty Acids (Grams per Serving)
Pound cake	4.3
Microwave popcorn (regular)	2.2
Margarine (stick)	1.8–3.5
Snack crackers	1.8–2.5
Vegetable shortening	1.4–4.2
Vanilla wafers	1.3
Chocolate chip cookies	1.2–2.7
French fries (fast food)	0.7–3.6
Margarine (tub, regular)	0.4–1.6
Doughnuts	0.3–3.8
Salad dressings (regular)	0.06–1.1
White bread	0.06–0.7
Ready-to-eat breakfast cereals	0.05–0.5
Chocolate candies	0.04–2.8
Vegetable oils	0.01–0.06
Snack chips	0–1.2

Fatty acid data from USDA food composition data, 1995

more fluid, making them liquid at room temperature and perfect for salads.

Like their friendly cousins, the polyunsaturated fats (PUFAs), MUFAs are best known for their ability to decrease blood cholesterol levels if part of a healthful diet and have also been found to contribute to glycemic control, helping to keep blood sugar stable. In addition, foods containing MUFAs are partnered up with a spectrum of insulin-stabilizing and heart-helping phytonutrients such as phenols, beta-sitosterol, and lutein to ally forces. In the next chapter we will discuss how compounds in foods team up to protect your health and bolster fertility, a phenomenon called *synergy*.

A recent study conducted at the University of Kuopio, Finland, examined the relationship between fatty acids in the blood and glucose metabolism. After a three-week, high-saturated-fat diet, thirty-one subjects with impaired glucose tolerance were put on a "mono" (primarily monounsaturated fats) or "poly" (primarily polyunsaturated fats) diet for eight weeks. The study found that those subjects with higher amounts of oleic acid—a monounsaturated from olive oil—and alpha-linolenic acid, an omega-3 fatty acid polyunsaturated—had the most improvement in fasting plasma glucose.

Evidence from the Mediterranean diet also supports this research showing that consumption of MUFA-rich olive oil helps to reduce inflammatory processes and may benefit weight loss. The Mediterranean diet consists of a wide variety of fruits and vegetables offering a spectrum of phytonutrients and healthy fats and proteins from nuts, seeds, and fish.

 Kitchen Prescription

Stock your kitchen with nuts, olive oil, and avocados to get the benefits of health-promoting MUFAs. Trade in your chips and pretzels for a MUFA-rich snack mix including air-popped popcorn and raw nuts.

The Friend: Polyunsaturated Fats (PUFAs)

The human body needs fatty acids and can make all but two of them: linolenic acid and linoleic acid. These fats must be supplied by the diet, hence the phrase *essential fatty acids*. Used by the body to maintain cell membranes and make hormonelike substances that regulate blood pressure, clotting, immune response, insulin function, and blood lipids, the PUFA side of the fat family gets special treatment for its good behavior and positive impact on health.

A 2004 study published in the *Journal of Clinical Endocrinology and Metabolism* examined the relationship between PUFAs in the diet and PCOS. The study concluded that getting more PUFAs in the diet significantly benefits metabolic and endocrine effects in women with PCOS.

Omega-3 Fatty Acids. Omega-3 fatty acids, also known as linolenic acid, are essential fatty acids (EFAs) that come from both plant and animal sources. Given linolenic acid, the body can make eicosapentaenoic acid (EPA) and docosahexaenoic acid (DHA), the two major fatty acids in fish. The greatest amounts of EPA and DHA are found in oily, dark-fleshed fish that live in deep, cold waters such as tuna, bluefish, and salmon. Alpha-linolenic acid is the other essential fatty acid and is found most abundantly in canola oil but also in flaxseed, walnuts, and soybeans, which contain a balance of omega-3 fats.

In human studies, omega-3 fatty acids have been shown to improve many of the negative effects of insulin resistance by lowering blood pressure and triglyceride concentrations that hamper the function of insulin-secreting cells. Additionally, studies have shown that omega-3s are of great importance in conception, successful pregnancy, and the health and intelligence of the unborn child.

A 2004 study published in *Obstetrics and Gynecological Survey* points to a number of benefits from omega-3 fatty acids in women dealing with infertility issues. The study suggests that omega-3s:

❖ Help to prevent and reverse menstrual problems (*dysmenor-rhea*) by reducing inflammation
❖ Increase the chances of becoming pregnant by increasing blood flow to the uterus
❖ Reduce the risk of premature birth
❖ Increase the length of pregnancy and birth weight
❖ Promote growth of the fetus by improving blood flow to the placenta
❖ May help to prevent preeclampsia, postpartum depression, menopausal problems, osteoporosis, and breast cancer

In 2004, the *Journal of the American Dietetic Association* reported that women with gestational diabetes mellitus have a greater risk of developing type 2 diabetes mellitus and suggested increasing PUFAs to reduce this risk. Similarly, a 2004 study published in *Lipids* found that women with gestational diabetes were consuming more saturated fats and less omega-3 fats. The study suggested to increase omega-3s to benefit pregnant women and stave off diabetes.

In addition, omega-3 fatty acids are capable of entering the brain, and research shows these essential fats have beneficial effects on the developing brain of the fetus and intelligence later in life. A 2005 study found that children whose mothers consumed docosahexaenoic acid (DHA) during pregnancy and lactation scored better in mental processing tests at age four.

Omega-6 Fatty Acids. Omega-6 fatty acids, also known as linoleic acid, are much more common in the American diet and are found in soybean oil, safflower oil, sunflower oil, corn oil, wheat germ, and sesame. While omega-6 fatty acids are healthy fats, there is a dark side to these characters that has been created by modern technology. Omega-6s, when left unbalanced by their anti-inflammatory counterpart (omega-3), can promote inflammation, possibly reducing the success of conception and pregnancy. They may also contribute to the development of diabetes and heart disease. Thus, researchers postulate that because omega-6 fatty acids are more readily available and consumed in Western countries, and that because our Paleolithic ancestors consumed a balance of omega-3 to omega-6 fatty acids, an imbalance could negatively influence inflammatory processes associated with insulin function, fertility, diabetes, and heart disease.

A 2005 study looked at PUFAs and the risk for preterm delivery. PUFAs affect levels of inflammatory prostaglandins, which affect many reproductive functions including ovulation. The study found that an imbalance of omega-6 to omega-3 fatty acids encourages preterm delivery.

Remember to strive for a good balance of omega-3 to omega-6. To get the maximum health benefits from the PUFAs, the ratio of omega-3 to omega-6 in our diet should be two to one, which can be achieved by consuming more whole foods and following some of our practical tips.

 Kitchen Prescription

To improve your ratio of omega-3 fatty acids to omega-6 fatty acids:

* ✤ Select walnuts as a snack.
* ✤ Look for new food products with enhanced omega-3s, including eggs (never raw during prepregnancy or pregnancy!), breads, frozen waffles, and cereals.
* ✤ Try flaxseed meal or hempseed meal as an addition to smoothies, cereals, and baked goods.
* ✤ Include cold-water cooked fish (like salmon) in your diet.

Culinary Caution: The Dish on Fish and Mercury. Although there is no doubt that including fish in your diet will deliver protective essential fatty acids and B vitamins, research shows that certain types of fish may contain dangerous levels of mercury. Nearly all fish and shellfish contain traces of methylmercury, a type of mercury found in water that can be harmful, especially to unborn babies and young children whose nervous systems are still developing. The risk for mercury lies in both the type of seafood consumed, as well as the amount. Through a joint consumer advisory, the FDA and the Environmental Protection Agency (EPA) warn that women who may be trying to become pregnant, pregnant women, nursing mothers, and young children should avoid the types of fish and shellfish with higher levels of mercury and eat only those that have lower levels.

If you regularly eat types of fish high in methylmercury, the substance can accumulate in your blood over time. Although it is removed from the body naturally, it may take more than a year for the levels to drop significantly, which is why women who are trying to become pregnant also should avoid eating certain types of fish.

While almost all fish and shellfish contain traces of methylmercury, larger fish that have lived longer contain the highest levels, as it has accumulated over time. Avoid eating shark, swordfish, or king mackerel because they contain high levels of mercury and pose the greatest risk. You should be eating up to twelve ounces (two average meals) a week of a variety of fish and shellfish that are lower in mercury. (We offer several recipes incorporating fish in Chapter 10.) Five of the most commonly eaten fish that are low in mercury are shrimp, canned light tuna, salmon, and catfish. In addition, albacore (white) tuna has more mercury than canned light tuna.

When choosing your meals of fish and shellfish, you may eat up to six ounces, one average meal, of albacore tuna per week. In addition, you should check to see if advisories exist concerning the safety of fish caught in local lakes, rivers, and coastal areas. If no advice is available, eat up to six ounces per week of fish you catch from local waters, but don't consume any other fish during that week.

Not All Carbs Are Created Equal

Carbohydrates are produced by photosynthesis in plants and are the primary source of energy found in plant foods including fruits, vegetables, grains, legumes, and tubers. Carbohydrates have an important role in the functioning of the internal organs, nervous system, and muscles and are the best source of energy for endurance athletes because they provide both an immediate and time-released energy source. These compounds are needed to regulate protein and fat metabolism, as well as help to fight infections, promote growth, and lubricate the joints.

Once grouped into two main categories, the simple carbs included sugars—such as fruit sugar (fructose), corn or grape sugar (dextrose or glucose), and table sugar (sucrose)—while complex carbs included everything made of three or more linked sugars. In the digestive system, carbohydrates are broken down into single sugar molecules that are then absorbed into the bloodstream and used as energy.

It's a shame that the entire carbohydrate family gets a bad rap for their delinquent stripped cousins. The naked truth of the matter is that when the integrity of whole grains is preserved, the effects on health are nothing short of wholesome.

Traditionally, it has been assumed that complex carbohydrates cause smaller rises in blood sugar than do simple carbohydrates. A growing body of evidence, however, contradicts this notion. In fact, white bread and potatoes are digested almost immediately to glucose, causing blood sugar to rapidly spike—refuting the theory that complex carbohydrates are different from simple sugars in terms of their effects on blood sugar levels.

The Glycemic Index Versus the Glycemic Load

A new system that had been embraced by many in the scientific community, called the *glycemic index* (*GI*), rates foods according to how fast and how high they push blood sugar, giving us a better indication of how carb-rich foods affect health. It has been shown that the GI of a food depends on the speed of digestion and absorption into the body, which is largely determined by both its physical and chemical properties. Typically, foods with less starch to gelatinize, or form a jelly (such as pasta), and those containing a high level of soluble fiber (such as whole-grain barley, oats, and rye) have slower rates of digestion and lower GI values.

Another important factor on GI values is the ratio of a compound called *amylose* to a fiber called *amylopectin*. Foods with a higher amylose-to-amylopectin ratio, such as legumes (beans, lentils, split peas) and parboiled rice (quick-cooking rice), tend to have lower GI values, because of the compact structure of amylase, which blunts how quickly the carbohydrate is broken down to its simplest form. Conversely, amylopectin is a branched compound—making it more available to enzymatic attack in the body—promoting digestion.

Use of the GI has shown that many complex carbohydrates (such as the white bread and potatoes noted) cause endocrine responses that rival pure glucose, further casting doubt on the usefulness of the simple versus complex classification system.

The principal argument against the GI concept is that it cannot tell the entire story, as blood sugar levels are influenced by both the quantity and the quality (GI rating) of the carbohydrate. In response to this concern, the concept of *glycemic load* (*GL*) was introduced. Defined as the product of the GI value of a food and its carbohydrate content, GL incorporates both the quality and quantity of carbohydrate consumed.

Dietary GL quantifies the glucose-raising potential of dietary carbohydrates. In general, carbohydrate-dense foods with low-fiber content have high GI and GL values—including potatoes, refined cereal products, and many sugar-sweetened beverages— whereas whole grains, fruits, and vegetables with high-fiber content provide low to very low GLs per serving. It should be noted, however, that many low-GI foods are not necessarily high in fiber (such as pasta, basmati rice, and dairy products), whereas some high-fiber, whole-meal bread and cereal products are high in GI.

Valuable research in recent years has offered additional insight into how carbohydrates affect our endocrine system, including insulin and inflammatory processes, as well as hunger, overeating, and weight gain.

Refined Versus Whole Carbohydrates

When it became common practice to refine the wheat flour for bread by milling it and discarding the bran and germ, consumers lost a myriad of health-protective nutrients. In the 1940s, Congress passed legislation requiring that all grain products that cross state lines be enriched with iron, thiamin, riboflavin, and niacin. In 1996, this legislation was amended to include folate, because of its important role in preventing birth defects. Although enrichment—the process of adding nutrients to a food to meet a specific standard—restores and raises many of the nutrients lost during refining, recent research shows that the health consequences cannot be compensated by adding individual nutrients back to a refined grain product for several reasons.

First, by removing the germ and bran layers of a grain, a naturally low-GI food is turned into a high-GI one. The fibrous coating serves to slow digestion, keeping blood sugar on an even keel. Also, the surface area is increased with refined grain products, enhancing digestive enzyme processes. As we discussed previously, this is an important element to keeping insulin levels low and maintaining a healthy weight—both important factors for ovulation.

Second, many nutrients in the germ and bran layers are not added back to the refined grain product, or the body poorly absorbs them. This is especially true of minerals, which are not as well absorbed from enriched foods as from naturally occurring sources. Three minerals in whole grains that may benefit fertility include:

* **Magnesium** for its important role in insulin function
* **Zinc** for its role in keeping leptin levels adequate to discourage weight gain and infertility as well as for a healthy immune system (as we noted in Chapter 2)
* **Selenium** for its insulin-mimicking effects and activity with antioxidant enzymes and benefit to sperm quality (which we'll discuss in Chapter 5)

Third, this "New Nutritional Frontier" is still in its infancy, and we have yet to identify all of the health-protective compounds in every food. When we alter a food from its natural state, by refining for example, we may be removing a cocktail of phytonutrients and other compounds that protect us from disease.

How Carbohydrate Choices Affect Your Weight

Because of their high-fiber and water content, whole-grain foods contain fewer calories gram for gram than the same amount of corresponding refined grain food. The Nurses' Health Study (NHS) showed that women with the greatest increase of intake of whole grains gained an average of 1.52 kilograms less than did those with the smallest increase in intake of whole-grain foods. In addition, women with the highest consumption of whole grains had a 49 percent lower risk of major weight gain than did women with the highest consumption of refined grains. Researchers believe that the insulin-elevating effects of high-GI foods promote weight gain by directing nutrients away from use in muscles and toward storage in fat cells.

Almost every study conducted on the effects of carbohydrates on appetite has shown that low-GI foods produce a feeling of satiety, or satisfaction, for a longer period of time than do their high-GI counterparts. One study found both lower levels of blood sugar and a slower return of hunger after meals with a bean-based dish (low GI) versus a potato dish (high GI).

How Carbohydrate Choices Affect PCOS and Insulin Issues

Because women with PCOS have higher levels of the appetite-regulating hormone ghrelin (as we discussed in Chapter 2), studies show they feel less satiated and hungry after a meal. Consuming foods that are low GI may promote satiety, keep insulin levels stable, and discourage weight gain—all important for ovulation.

The Framingham Research Study conducted at the Jean Mayer U.S. Department of Agriculture, Human Nutrition Research Center on Aging at Tufts University examined the relationship between whole grains and metabolic risk factors for type 2 diabetes and cardiovascular disease. Using 2,941 participants, the study found an inverse association between whole-grain intake and fasting insulin, specifically among overweight participants.

A Harvard study looked at the intake of whole versus refined grains among 75,521 women free of diabetes and heart disease. The study determined that the women who included the most whole grains into their diet substantially reduced the risk of diabetes, especially among women with a body mass index (BMI) greater than 25.

A study conducted at the University of Minnesota had similar findings. This study examined the relationship between carbohydrates, fiber, magnesium, and the glycemic index with the incidence of diabetes among 35,988 Iowa women. The study concluded that whole grains, cereal fiber, and dietary magnesium have a protective role in the development of diabetes.

The Insulin Resistance Atherosclerosis Study (IRAS) evaluated specific dietary patterns and their relationship with insulin resistance and found those participants consuming the most whole grains, specifically in the form of dark breads, had increased insulin sensitivity. Researchers believe the fiber and magnesium found in whole grains may be to credit for the beneficial effects on insulin function.

Carbs in the Kitchen

Now that we've set the stage for understanding how carbohydrates affect insulin levels, let's put it into practice! Here we offer information on classifying carbs, show you how easy it is to clean up your carb act, and give you practical pairings to get your healthy carbs and healthy fats, deliciously.

While certain fruits, such as watermelon and carrots, are high on the GI scale (as seen in Table 3.2), they should not be avoided because of their abundance of phytonutrients, fiber, and other nutrients. However, aim to stock your pantry with moderate- (Table 3.3, page 52) and low-GI foods (Table 3.4, page 53) and enjoy them often.

Small changes can make a big impact on your health. The following list offers some helpful suggestions for replacing the carbs higher on the glycemic index with some lower alternatives.

* Instead of white bread try dark, whole-grain breads. Pepperidge Farm makes a line of whole-grain breads that contain no trans fats.
* Instead of white rice, try brown rice, brown basmati rice, or wild rice.

TABLE 3.2 **High-GI Foods (>69)**	
Product	**Food**
Breads and bakery	White bread
	Pretzels
	French bread
Breakfast cereals	Cornflakes
	Rice Krispies
	Cheerios
Confectionery	Jelly beans
	Life Savers
	Skittles
Fruits and vegetables	Carrots
	Watermelon
	Potatoes
	Parsnips
Rice, grains, and pastas	Low-amylase rice

✤ Instead of sugary breakfast cereal try steel-cut oats or low-added-sugar bran cereal.

✤ Instead of pretzels try air-popped popcorn.

✤ Instead of potatoes try beans or whole-grain pasta.

✤ Instead of white crackers try whole-grain rye or wheat crackers.

✤ Instead of cakes, light muffins, or pastries try low-fat bran muffins or use whole-grain mixes.

In addition, here are some ideas from Healing Gourmet on getting a daily dose of those healthy fats and carbs without sacri-

TABLE 3.3 **Moderate-GI Foods (55–69)**	
Product	**Food**
Breads and bakery	Sourdough
	Pita bread
	Barley bread
	Rye bread
	Whole-wheat bread
Breakfast cereals	Quick-cooking oatmeal
	Cream of wheat
	Muesli
Fruits and vegetables	Pineapple
	Banana
Rice, grains, and pastas	Brown rice
	Linguine
	White rice
	Popcorn

ficing taste! For more ideas, see the recipe and meal planning sections, and visit our website at healinggourmet.com.

* Kashi Go Lean Waffle with all-natural peanut butter for whole grains, PUFAs, and low-GI legumes
* Ryvita Dark Rye crackers and hummus for whole grains, low-GI legumes, and MUFAs
* Grilled wild salmon and brown rice for omega-3s and whole grains
* Stonyfield Farms Black Cherry Yogurt and ground flax for low-GI carbs and omega-3s

TABLE 3.4 **Low-GI Foods (<55)**	
Product	**Food**
Breads and bakery	Pumpernickel
	Heavy mixed grain
Breakfast cereals	All Bran
	Toasted muesli
	Psyllium-based cereal
	Oatmeal (old-fashioned)
Dairy foods	Soy milk
	Milk, skim
	Yogurt, low-fat, fruit
Fruits and vegetables	Grapefruit
	Peaches
	Apples
	Pears
	Oranges
	Grapes
	Kiwis
	Sweet potatoes
Rice, grains, and pastas	Fettuccini
	Whole-wheat spaghetti
	Spaghetti
	Long-grain rice
	Bulgur
Legumes	Peanuts
	Soybeans
	Lentils
	Chickpeas
	Baked beans (canned)

Feast on Fiber: Bulk Is Better

One of the insulin-balancing properties of whole-grain, carbohydrate-rich foods is their abundance of fiber—an important non-nutritive compound for health that helps to keep blood sugar balanced, promotes a healthy weight, and sweeps cholesterol out of the body.

There are two general categories of fiber: *insoluble* and *soluble*. There are several types of insoluble fibers. *Cellulose* can be found in cabbage, peas, apples, root vegetables, whole-wheat flour, beans, bran, and wheat. *Hemicellulose* is found in bran, cereals, and whole grains. *Lignan*, most abundantly found in omega-3-rich flaxseed, is a phytonutrient that works very much like an insoluble fiber. Fiber is actually classified as a carbohydrate, and in the United States the total carbohydrates listed on a food label will include dietary fiber—although it is listed separately. Insoluble fiber is also important to regulate gastrointestinal functions and to keep the colon clean.

Research studies confirm, and it is the position of the American Dietetic Association, that fiber is an important element in stabilizing blood sugar, reducing cholesterol, achieving a healthy weight, and preventing heart disease. Water-soluble fiber, in particular, is beneficial for several key reasons.

* It slows digestion and the absorption of nutrients, resulting in a slow and steady release of glucose from the other carbohydrates that accompany it.
* It delays stomach emptying, causing a feeling of fullness or satiety that is useful in achieving or maintaining a healthy weight.
* It soaks up excess bile acids found in the intestinal tract, which are converted into blood cholesterol by the body.

Soluble fibers can be divided into three major types: *pectins* (found in root vegetables, cabbage, apples, whole-wheat bran, and beans), *gums* (which can be obtained from oatmeal, dried beans, and other legumes), and *mucilages* (which are synthesized by plant cells and are found in food additives).

Fiber, Insulin Levels, and Weight Gain

Harvard studies, the Nurses' Health Study, and the Health Professionals Follow-Up Study found that a diet low in cereal fiber and rich in high-GI foods (which cause big spikes in blood sugar) more than doubled the risk of type 2 diabetes when compared to a diet high in cereal fiber and low in high-GI foods. Another Harvard study found that weight gain among 74,091 nurses was inversely associated with high-fiber, whole-grain foods and positively associated with the intake of refined-grain foods.

Getting the Most Fiber into Your Diet

New fiber guidelines recommend women under fifty consume 28 or more grams of fiber per day, and women over fifty consume 25 or more grams of fiber daily. Clinical studies have shown that up to 50 grams of fiber per day can improve glycemic control as well as reduce lipid levels. In Table 3.5, we summarize some general sources of fiber. Remember to increase the amount of both kinds of fiber. Here are some tips to help you get a good balance.

- ❖ Choose fresh fruits or vegetables rather than juice.
- ❖ Eat the skin and membranes of cleaned fruits and vegetables.
- ❖ Choose bran and whole-grain breads and cereals daily.
- ❖ When you increase fiber, you should also increase your water intake.

TABLE 3.5 **Fiber Content of Selected Foods**

Food Item	Total(g)	Soluble(g)	Insoluble(g)
Legumes			
Pinto beans (½ cup, cooked)	7.4	1.9	5.5
Chickpeas (½ cup)	6.2	1.3	4.9
Kidney beans (½ cup, cooked)	5.8	2.9	2.9
Navy beans (½ cup, cooked)	5.8	2.2	3.6
Northern beans (½ cup)	5.6	1.4	4.2
Soybeans (½ cup, cooked)	5.1	2.3	2.8
Tofu (½ cup)	1.4	0.9	0.6
Cereal Grains			
Barley (½ cup, cooked)	4.2	0.9	3.3
Millet (½ cup, cooked)	3.3	0.6	2.7
Bulgur (½ cup, cooked)	2.9	0.5	2.4
Noodles (whole-wheat)	2.3	0.5	1.8
Rice, brown (½ cup, cooked)	1.7	0.1	1.6
Rice, wild (½ cup, cooked)	1.5	0.2	1.3
Couscous (½ cup, cooked)	1.3	0.3	1.0

Noodles (white spaghetti)	0.9	0.4	0.5
Noodles (spinach, ½ cup)	0.9	0.4	0.5
Rice, white (½ cup, cooked)	0.2	0	0.2
Breads (1 medium slice)			
Pita (7″ diameter, wheat)	4.4	0.7	3.7
Whole-wheat	1.9	0.3	1.6
Multigrain	1.8	0.3	1.5
Pumpernickel	1.5	0.8	0.7
Rye	1.5	0.8	0.7
Tortilla (6″ diameter, plain)	1.4	0.2	1.1
Tortilla (8″ diameter, plain)	1.4	0.4	1.0
White or sourdough	0.7	0.4	0.3
Cereal (1 cup)			
All Bran	10.0	1.0	9.0
Raisin bran	8.4	1.2	7.2
Oatmeal	3.8	1.8	2.0
Cherrios	2.6	1.2	1.4

(continued)

TABLE 3.5 *(continued)*

Food Item	Total(g)	Soluble(g)	Insoluble(g)
Cereal *(continued)*			
Farina	1.2	0.5	0.7
Cornflakes	0.7	0	0.7
Grits, corn	0.4	0	0.4
Snacks			
Popcorn (microwave, 3 cups)	2.4	0	2.4
Popcorn (light, 3 cups)	2.3	0	2.3
Fruits (fresh)			
Apple (3" diameter)	5.7	1.5	4.2
Figs (3 small)	5.3	2.3	3.0
Orange (3" diameter)	4.4	2.6	1.8
Raspberries (½ cup)	4.2	0.4	3.8
Pear (3" diameter)	4.0	2.2	1.8
Blackberries (½ cup)	3.8	3.1	0.7
Mango (medium)	3.7	1.5	2.2
Peach (medium)	3.2	1.3	1.9

Kiwi (large)	2.4	0.7	3.1
Banana (7" long)	2.1	0.7	2.8
Prunes (3 medium)	0.9	1.0	1.9
Blueberries (½ cup)	1.7	0.2	1.9
Strawberries (½ cup)	1.4	0.5	1.9
Plum (large)	0.8	0.9	1.7
Cherries (½ cup, fresh)	1.2	0.5	1.7
Applesauce (½ cup)	1.1	0.5	1.6
Raisins (¼ cup)	1.1	0.4	1.5
Grapefruit (half, 4" diameter)	0.3	1.2	1.5
Pineapple (½ cup)	0.9	0.1	1.0
Grapes (½ cup)	0.5	0.3	0.8
Melon (⅕ of 6" diameter)	0.5	0.2	0.7
Juice (orange, 6 oz)	0.2	0.2	0.4
Juice (apple, 6 oz)	0.1	0.1	0.2
Vegetables			
Artichoke (medium, cooked)	1.8	4.7	6.5
Brussels sprouts (½ cup)	1.3	2.0	3.3

(continued)

TABLE 3.5 *(continued)*

Food Item	Total(g)	Soluble(g)	Insoluble(g)
Vegetables (continued)			
Jicama (raw, ½ cup)	3.2	1.7	1.5
Chilies (hot pepper, raw)	3.0	1.5	1.5
Carrots (baby, 6)	2.8	1.4	1.4
Corn (½ cup)	2.0	0.3	1.7
Beans (cooked, ½ cup)	1.9	0.8	1.1
Cabbage (green, cooked)	1.8	0.8	1.0
Cauliflower (½ cup)	1.7	0.4	1.3
Carrots (cooked, ½ cup)	1.6	1.1	1.5
Beets (½ cup)	1.5	0.7	0.8
Asparagus spears (cooked)	1.4	0.7	0.7
Bok choy (½ cup)	1.4	0.5	0.9
Broccoli (cooked)	1.4	1.2	1.2
Eggplant, cooked (½ cup)	1.3	0.4	0.9
Cauliflower (raw, ½ cup)	1.3	0.5	0.8
Broccoli (raw, ½ cup)	1.3	0.5	0.8
Celery (1 large stalk)	1.1	0.4	0.7

Lettuce (romaine, 1 cup)	0.9	0.3	0.6
Lettuce (iceberg, 1 cup)	0.8	0.1	0.7
Cabbage (red, shredded)	0.8	0.3	0.5
Greens (cooked, ½ cup)	0.4	0.1	0.3
Frozen and Mixed Vegetables (½ cup)			
Lima beans/corn	4.9	1.8	3.1
Peas (cooked, ½ cup)	4.3	1.2	3.1
Corn/green beans/carrots	4.0	1.9	2.1
Sweet potatoes (½ cup)	3.8	1.4	2.4
Pumpkin (mashed, ½ cup)	3.6	0.5	3.1
Squash (winter, ½ cup cooked)	3.3	1.9	1.4
Potato (w/skin, medium)	2.9	1.2	1.7
Spinach (cooked, ½ cup)	2.7	0.5	2.2
Peas/carrots	2.5	0.9	1.6
Onions (½ cup cooked)	2.0	1.2	0.8
Broccoli/peppers/mushrooms	1.8	0.7	1.1
Mushrooms (cooked, sliced)	1.8	0.2	1.6
Squash (butternut, ½ cup)	1.7	0.7	1.0

(continued)

TABLE 3.5 *(continued)*

Food Item	Total(g)	Soluble(g)	Insoluble(g)
Frozen and Mixed Vegetables (½ cup) *(continued)*			
Potato (mashed, ½ cup)	1.6	0.9	0.7
Broccoli/cauliflower	1.5	0.6	0.9
Peppers (green/red, ½ cup)	1.3	0.5	0.8
Water chestnuts (½ cup)	1.2	0.9	1.3
Zucchini (cooked, ½ cup)	1.2	0.5	0.7
Tomatoes (medium, raw)	0.9	0	0.9
Spinach (raw, 1 cup)	0.4	0.1	0.3

✤ Eat fewer processed foods and more fresh ones, as processing often removes fiber.

✤ Try to get fiber from foods rather than fiber supplements, as foods are more nutritious and supply an array of health-promoting phytonutrients.

Love Your Legumes

Beans not only benefit insulin levels and promote a healthy weight but also deliver a baby-boosting dose of calcium and folate, plus protein and fiber. The case for beans is so strong we're devoting this section to these bundles of joy!

Beans release sugar slowly into the bloodstream, ensuring blood sugar stays stable. The insoluble fiber causes the body to produce more insulin receptor sites—tiny "docks" that insulin molecules latch onto—meaning more insulin gets into cells where it is needed and less is present in the bloodstream where it can cause problems. The low GI of beans has been attributed to many factors including their fiber, tannin, and phytic acid contents.

Phytoestrogens, found in legumes, have been found to improve glucose control and insulin resistance, as well as reduce cholesterol. Researchers believe these compounds modulate the secretion of insulin from the pancreas and also act as antioxidants.

 Kitchen Prescription

Try our recipe for Maternity Minestrone in Chapter 10. It's filled with kidney and cannellini beans that will fill you up without weighing you down. In the mood for Mexican? Try our Enchilada Casserole, chock-full of black and pinto beans. Bean up!

The folate in beans is critical in prenatal nutrition for the proper development of a baby's brain and spinal cord, so too is the calcium for strong bones and teeth. Beans also provide iron to help prevent anemia. See Chapter 7 for more on these nutrients in prenatal nutrition.

Now that you have some ideas for balancing the healthy and unhealthy fats and carbohydrates, plus getting a healthy dose of fiber and learning to love your legumes, it's time to look at the benefits of increasing your intake of antioxidants and phytonutrients, as well as how to incorporate these important foods into your fertility-boosting diet.

4

Antioxidants, Phytonutrients, and Other Fertility-Boosting Nutrients

RESEARCH SHOWS THAT individual compounds in foods work together to help balance blood sugar, reduce inflammation, quell appetite, and prepare a woman's body for a successful pregnancy. Like musical notes, each adds a unique element to the symphony of your health, not just in boosting fertility, but also helping to stave off diabetes, heart disease, cancer, and many other chronic diseases. However, just as the quarterback alone can't win the game, no single nutrient has the ability to conquer disease. In this chapter, we'll discuss the synergistic relationship of nutrients in foods as the keys to a fertility-boosting nutritional strategy.

Free Radical Defense

Free radicals make about ten thousand attacks every day on the cells in our body. These unstable oxygen molecules have lost an electron and move swiftly, stealing electrons from other molecules. This process in turn creates more free radicals and leaves damaged cells in the wake. Some free radicals arise normally during metabolism, but environmental factors such as pollution, poor food choices, radiation, cigarette smoke, and herbicides can also generate free radicals.

Our body's defense—including our immune system and antioxidants produced by the liver (such as glutathione and super-oxide dismutase)—needs fuel from outside sources to conquer our health-robbing adversary. Quite simply, the fuel is food, and good dietary decisions tip the odds in favor of increasing fertility and preventing disease.

Quest for Fertility: An Increased Need to Fight Free Radicals

Hyperglycemia, or high blood sugar, is a factor associated with PCOS and is known to cause free radical damage (or oxidative stress). Research shows that balancing blood sugar and incorporating antioxidants into the diet may help to reduce oxidant stress. Free radicals have been found to have detrimental effects on the function of many cells including:

* Insulin-secreting beta cells of the pancreas
* Fat cells
* Muscle cells
* Nerve cells
* Sex (or germ) cells

Each nutrient and antioxidant plays a special role in protecting cells and organs from oxidative damage. Therefore, it's important to include the full spectrum in your diet to tip the odds in favor of boosting health and fertility. Let's take a look at some of the superstars you should be incorporating into your diet every day.

The Antioxidant Superstars

With the evolution of technology, researchers are able to measure the levels of antioxidants in specific foods, helping us to identify the star players. Digestion, absorption, and methods of cooking play a role in the amount of antioxidants in foods, so be sure to change it up and keep your diet varied. Table 4.1 summarizes the top twenty food sources of antioxidants. You'll learn about the phytonutrients responsible for these free radical fighting actions in the next section.

 Kitchen Prescription

Many factors affect the levels of antioxidants in foods, including the method of cooking. Some antioxidants, such as vitamin C, are water soluble; others, such as lycopene and other carotenoids, are lipid or fat soluble. In general, lipid-soluble antioxidants are best absorbed by the body when cooked and consumed with a bit of fat (oil); whereas water-soluble foods are best fresh, as cooking destroys these compounds or they are lost in the water.

Phytonutrient Fuel: A Clean Pass

Much of the good press antioxidants get is due to tiny compounds called *phytonutrients* found inside fruits, vegetables, legumes, and grains. These phytonutrients (*phyto* meaning plant) protect plants against harsh weather conditions and hungry insects; they even heal the wounds made by the nibbling moth. With their own defensive lineup, plant foods stand ready to guard against hungry predators, trying to take a bite, or fungi that hang around, draining their resources.

TABLE 4.1 **Top Twenty Food Sources of Antioxidants**

Rank	Food	Serving Size	Total Antioxidant Capacity per Serving
1	Small red beans (dried)	Half cup	13,727
2	Wild blueberries	1 cup	13,427
3	Red kidney beans (dried)	Half cup	13,259
4	Pinto beans	Half cup	11,864
5	Blueberries (cultivated)	1 cup	9,019
6	Cranberries	1 cup (whole)	8,983
7	Artichokes (cooked)	1 cup (hearts)	7,904
8	Blackberries	1 cup	7,701
9	Dried prunes	Half cup	7,291
10	Raspberries	1 cup	6,058
11	Strawberries	1 cup	5,938
12	Red Delicious apples	One	5,900
13	Granny Smith apples	One	5,381
14	Pecans	1 ounce	5,095
15	Sweet cherries	1 cup	4,873
16	Black plums	One	4,844
17	Russet potatoes (cooked)	One	4,649
18	Black beans (dried)	Half cup	4,181
19	Plums	One	4,118
20	Gala apples	One	3,903

This plant protection system—essentially antioxidants and phytonutrients—not only serves as defense but is also credited for the vibrant colors and delicious flavors of our food. Interestingly, distinguishing colors is a trait common only to humans and a few species of primates. So the foods most appealing to our eye are also most appealing to our body to prevent and treat diseases.

It should come as no surprise that fruits and vegetables with higher levels of antioxidants produce fresher food for longer periods of time (or shelf life) with less risk of mold. These foods are better equipped to preserve and protect themselves; and when we take a bite, those antioxidants and phytonutrients are passed along to us.

Unfortunately, the development of agriculture some ten thousand years ago caused a shift away from our diverse plant-based diet that provides a spectrum of essential vitamins and minerals, and tens of thousands of protective phytonutrients. Replacing this delicious and defensive diet with processed foods, refined grains, and added oils, sugar, and salt has led to the rise of chronic diseases including diabetes, heart disease, and cancer, and possibly the rising rates of infertility. In fact, today most Americans eat between two and three servings of fruits and vegetables per day (when the optimum is seven to nine servings), and a minority eat none at all.

Advances in technology have allowed us to further explore compounds in foods on a molecular level, distinguishing between the thousands of plant nutrients in individual foods and food families. This "new nutritional frontier" provides us with critical information on how best we can use foods to balance blood sugar, prevent inflammation, and achieve optimum health in preparation for pregnancy. It is estimated that twenty-five thousand individual phytonutrients have been identified in fruits, vegetables, and grains; a large percentage still remain unknown and need to be identified before we can fully understand their health benefits. Let's take a look at the lineup.

The Vitamin and Mineral Team of Players

These "old school" standbys have taught us few new things in recent decades. Although we have known about the actions of vitamins and minerals and requirements *during* pregnancy for some time, only recently have we begun to understand their individual roles in facilitating fertility and preventing disease. We offer information on the vitamins and minerals as a percentage of the daily value (DV). Talk with your registered dietitian to meet your personal nutritional needs.

Biotin

It has been known for many years that a biotin deficiency causes an improper use of glucose in the body. In laboratory studies, biotin has been found to stimulate the secretion of insulin, helping to reduce blood sugar—a key factor in PCOS and the development of gestational diabetes.

 Healing Tip

Those low-GI, carb-rich foods we talked about in Chapter 3 supply sugar-balancing biotin. While there is no recommended daily allowance (RDA) for biotin, you can get it in soybeans, rice bran, peanut butter, barley, and oatmeal.

Calcium

Like magnesium, calcium helps cells to communicate with one another and plays a role in mediating the constriction and relaxation of blood vessels, nerve impulse transmission, muscle contraction, and the secretion of hormones, including insulin. This common mineral has beneficial effects on lipids and may aid in weight control as well. By forming insoluble soaps with fatty acids in the intestine, calcium helps to prevent the absorption of part of the dietary fat, thus reducing cholesterol. Calcium is also critical in the development of your future child's bones and teeth.

 Healing Tip

Get calcium in low-fat yogurt (415 mg or 42 percent DV), skim milk (402 mg or 30 percent DV), tofu (204 mg or 20 percent DV), orange juice (200 mg or 20 percent DV), salmon (181 mg or 18 percent DV), cooked spinach (120 mg or 12 percent DV), kale (94 mg or 9 percent DV), and bok choy (74 mg or 7 percent DV).

Calculating Calcium. The following foods provide the same amount of calcium. Eat a variety of calcium-rich foods to maximize your absorption of this important mineral. Visit the Office of Dietary Supplements at http://ods.od.nih.gov/factsheets/calcium.asp to learn more.

8 ounces of milk = 1 cup of yogurt = 1½ ounces of cheddar cheese = 1½ cups of cooked kale = 2¼ cups of cooked broccoli = 8 cups of cooked spinach.

Folate

Folate gets its name from the Latin word *folium* for leaf, and hence is present in good amounts in leafy greens. Research shows that folate, working in conjunction with vitamin B_6 and vitamin B_{12}, helps to reduce levels of heart-harming homocysteine (Hcy). The results of more than eighty studies indicate that even moderately elevated levels of Hcy in the blood increase the risk of cardiovascular diseases. Because women with PCOS have an increased risk of heart disease, getting enough of these vitamins may help reduce risk. Folate is also very important to prevent neural tube defects, which we'll discuss in greater detail in Chapter 7.

 Healing Tip

Beans and Greens! If you frequently dine on beans and greens, you're fine with folate. You can get it in black-eyed peas (105 mcg or 25 percent DV), cooked spinach (100 mcg or 25 percent DV), great northern beans (90 mcg or 20 percent DV), asparagus (85 mcg or 20 percent DV), wheat germ (40 mcg or 10 percent DV), orange juice (35 mcg or 10 percent DV), peas (50 mcg or 15 percent DV), cooked broccoli (45 mcg or 15 percent DV), avocados (45 mcg or 10 percent DV), and peanuts (40 mcg or 10 percent DV).

Magnesium

As one of the most abundant ions present in living cells, studies have shown that magnesium helps insulin get inside cells and improve their function. When there is a low concentration of magnesium inside cells, insulin receptors don't function as well, worsening insulin resistance. It is also important for heart health, an increased risk factor for those suffering from PCOS.

Healing Tip

Magnificent Magnesium! Get it in a typical serving of halibut (90 mg or 20 percent DV), almonds (80 mg or 20 percent DV), cashews (75 mg or 20 percent DV), soybeans (75 mg or 20 percent DV), spinach (75 mg or 20 percent DV), oatmeal (55 mg or 15 percent DV), potatoes (50 mg or 15 percent DV), peanuts (50 mg or 15 percent DV), black-eyed peas (45 mg or 10 percent DV), yogurt (45 mg or 10 percent DV), baked beans (40 mg or 10 percent DV), and brown rice (40 mg or 10 percent DV).

Selenium

Although selenium is a mineral rather than a nutrient, it is a component of antioxidant enzymes. Selenium helps to protect cells against the effects of free radicals produced during normal metabolism. A recent study found an inverse relationship with selenium (as well as zinc) in the diet and the risk for gestational hyperglycemia.

Healing Tip

An average serving of Brazil nuts contains large quantities of selenium (540 mg or 780 percent DV). You can also find it in tuna (63 mg or 95 percent DV), cod (32 mg or 45 percent DV), turkey (32 mg or 45 percent DV), chicken (20 mg or 30 percent DV), noodles (17 mg or 25 percent DV), and oatmeal (12 mg or 15 percent DV).

Vitamin B₁ (Thiamin)

Vitamin B₁, or thiamin, is necessary for processing carbohydrates, fats, and protein, as well as the production of *adenine triphosphate* (*ATP*), the basic unit of energy in the body. Having an important role in nerve functioning, thiamin is also an important coenzyme that assists in the metabolism of glucose.

 Healing Tip

Get thiamin in lentils (0.17 mg or 15 percent DV), peas (0.19 mg or 17 percent DV), brown rice (0.10 mg or 9 percent DV), Brazil nuts (0.17 mg or 15 percent DV), pecans (0.13 mg or 12 percent DV), spinach (0.02 or 2 percent DV), medium oranges (0.05 mg or 5 percent DV), cantaloupes (0.07 mg or 6 percent DV).

Vitamin B₃ (Niacin)

Vitamin B₃, or niacin, is part of the *glucose tolerance factor* (*GTF*), which is important in keeping your body sensitive to insulin. A deficiency of niacin makes it difficult for your body to produce GTF, which could lead to or worsen insulin resistance.

 Healing Tip

Get niacin in chicken (9.52 mg or 68 percent DV), turkey (5.41 mg or 39 percent DV), salmon (6.68 mg or 48 percent DV), mackerel (5.83 mg or 42 percent DV), tuna (8.96 mg or 64 percent DV), barley (1.62 mg or 12 percent DV), bulgur (0.91 mg or 6 percent DV), pasta (1.56 mg or 11 percent DV), lentils (1.05 mg or 8 percent DV), dried peaches (3.5 mg or 3 percent DV), and avocados (0.63 or 4 percent DV).

Vitamin B₆

Vitamin B₆ is needed for more than one hundred enzymes involved in protein metabolism for support of the nervous and immune systems, to make hemoglobin, and to increase the oxygen it carries. It also helps maintain blood sugar within a normal range. A vitamin B₆ deficiency can result in a form of anemia that is similar to iron deficiency anemia, commonly seen in pregnancy. As mentioned earlier, vitamins B₆ and B₁₂ working in conjunction with folate help reduce levels of heart-harming homocysteine (Hcy).

Healing Tip

Boost Your Bs! You can find vitamin B₆ in a typical serving of potatoes (0.7 mg or 35 percent DV), garbanzo beans (0.57 mg or 30 percent DV), chicken breast (0.52 mg or 25 percent DV), oatmeal (0.42 mg or 20 percent DV), trout (0.29 mg or 15 percent DV), sunflower seeds (0.23 mg or 10 percent DV), avocados (0.20 mg or 10 percent DV), tuna (0.18 mg or 10 percent DV), and cooked spinach (0.14 mg or 8 percent DV).

Vitamin B₁₂

Vitamin B₁₂ helps maintain healthy nerve cells and red blood cells and is needed to manufacture DNA, the genetic material in all cells. Because vitamin B₁₂ is bound to the protein in food, it is found most abundantly in animal products. Like vitamin B₆ and folate, vitamin B₁₂ helps to reduce levels of heart-harming homocysteine (Hcy). In addition, a vitamin B₁₂ deficiency can cause pernicious anemia, as well as neurological damage in babies and adults. Because of this, women following a strict vegetarian diet should talk with their doctor and registered dietitian to make sure they are getting enough of this essential vitamin in their diet. If you are a vegetarian, speak with your doctor or dietitian about supplementing vitamin B$_{12}$, which is obtained primarily from animal sources.

Healing Tip

Go Fish! Vitamin B$_{12}$ is found in clams (84.1 mcg or 1,400 percent DV), trout (5.4 mcg or 90 percent DV), salmon (4.9 mcg or 80 percent DV), yogurt (1.4 mcg or 25 percent DV), tuna (1 mcg or 15 percent DV), and milk (0.9 mcg or 15 percent DV).

Vitamin C (Ascorbic Acid)

Vitamin C, or ascorbic acid, is a water-soluble vitamin. As we discussed earlier in the chapter, antioxidant nutrients have important roles in reducing free radical damage that is associated with hyperglycemia and PCOS, as well as in helping to prevent preeclampsia.

Healing Tip

Orange You Healthy? Get your daily dose of vitamin C in oranges (78 mg or 104 percent DV), grapefruit (132 mg or 178 percent DV), blueberries (14 mg or 19 percent DV), strawberries (122 mg or 163 percent DV), mangoes (57 mg or 76 percent DV), papaya (94 or 125 percent DV), cantaloupe (70 or 93 percent DV), watermelon (12 mg or 16 percent DV), sweet potatoes (18 mg or 24 percent DV), green peppers (95 mg or 125 percent DV), and red peppers (226 mg or 301 percent DV).

Vitamin E (Alpha-Tocopherol)

As a fat-soluble antioxidant vitamin, like vitamin C, vitamin E may protect against the free radical damage associated with hyperglycemia and PCOS. It may also help to reduce the risk of preeclampsia by reducing the oxidative stress caused by inflammatory cytokines, which can negatively affect the placenta.

 Healing Tip

Es to Please! Get it in wheat germ oil (20.3 mg or 100 percent DV), almonds (7.4 mg or 40 percent DV), sunflower seeds (6 mg or 30 percent DV), sunflower oil (5.6 mg or 30 percent DV), safflower oil (4.6 mg or 25 percent DV), hazelnuts (4.3 mg or 20 percent DV), peanut butter (4.2 mg or 20 percent DV), peanuts (2.2 mg or 10 percent DV), spinach (1.6 mg or 6 percent DV), broccoli (1.2 or 6 percent DV), soybean oil (1.3 mg or 6 percent DV), kiwis (1.1 mg or 6 percent DV), and mangoes (0.9 mg or 6 percent DV).

Zinc

Zinc is an essential mineral that is found in almost every cell. It stimulates the activity of approximately one hundred enzymes, which are substances that promote biochemical reactions in your body. It supports a healthy immune system, is needed for wound healing, and helps maintain your sense of taste and smell. It is also required for DNA synthesis and to support normal growth and development during pregnancy, childhood, and adolescence. A zinc deficiency reduces leptin, which, as we discussed in Chapter 2, helps to suppress appetite and prevent weight gain and obesity. According to a 2005 study published in *Nutrition*, zinc also plays an important role in stabilizing blood sugar and in reducing the risk of gestational hyperglycemia.

Healing Tip

Get zinc in oysters (16 mg or 100 percent DV), ready-to-eat break-fast cereal fortified with zinc (15 mg or 100 percent DV), low-fat yogurt (2.2 mg or 15 percent DV), baked beans (1.7 mg or 10 percent DV), cashews (1.6 mg or 10 percent DV), pecans (1.4 mg or 10 percent DV), chickpeas (1.3 mg or 8 percent DV), almonds (1 mg or 6 percent DV), walnuts (1 mg or 6 percent DV), chicken (1 mg or 6 percent DV), and cheese (1 mg or 6 percent DV).

The Phytonutrient Team of Players That Help with Fertility

Don't let the big names of these tiny compounds scare you. They deliver a powerful punch even when you don't call them by name. To boost fertility, it's important for a woman to include the full spectrum into her diet every day!

Phenolic Phytonutrients and Flavonoids

Phenolics represent a very large category of more than two thousand phytonutrients. The term *phenol* comes from the chemical structure of these phytonutrients that vary from having one to several powerful phenol groups, which have the ability to sweep up many free radicals as they circulate through the bloodstream. This reduces damage to cells and oxidation of LDL cholesterol. Considered to be some of the most powerful antioxidants, phenolics are being studied for their ability to slow the aging process and also have anti-inflammatory, heart-protective, and clot-busting effects. Let's take a look at the phenolic family and how each member allies forces for your health.

Flavonoids are molecular compounds found only in plants that serve as a defense mechanism. Because plants don't have the fight-or-flight option that animals do, they must protect themselves chemically; flavonoids make the plant tissue unappetizing to fungi, insects, and other organisms harmful to plants. Every plant makes flavonoids, but they tend to be concentrated in the leaves and fruit. Therefore, fruits tend to be a richer source of flavonoids than many vegetables. Dietary flavonoids have been found to repair a range of oxidative radical damages on DNA, which can contribute to disease and the ravages of aging.

 Healing Tip

Fabulous flavonoids can be found in apples, broccoli, celery, citrus fruits, cocoa, eggplants, endive, grapes, grapefruit, leeks, onion, parsley, raspberries, red wine (not advisable for women trying to get pregnant!), strawberries, and decaffeinated tea.

Anthocyanins. These brightly colored compounds have recently been found to have beneficial effects on fat cells by reducing their secretion of inflammatory cytokines. As we discussed in Chapter 2, cytokines like C-reactive protein have negative effects on insulin resistance and PCOS, as well as diabetes and heart disease.

 Healing Tip

Berry Delicious Medicine! You can find these compounds most readily in red-blue fruits, including blueberries, raspberries, lingonberries, cherries, currants, pomegranates, strawberries, concord grapes, cranberries, and elderberries. Buy them frozen, and add to smoothies or thaw for a quick addition to cereal.

Lignans. As a phytoestrogen, lignans have antioxidant action and have been found to facilitate weight loss and contribute to insulin control.

 Kitchen Prescription

Get the Flax! Lignans are found in high concentrations in flaxseed and olive oil as well as in legumes including peas, beans, and lentils. To get the maximum benefit of lignans, buy whole flaxseed, grind them in a coffee grinder, refrigerate, and eat what you grind within a few days. Sprinkle over cereal or yogurt, add to smoothies, or bake into whole-grain baked goods.

Carotenoid Phytonutrients

Carotenoids, a group of more than six hundred related nutrients, have received substantial attention both because of their provitamin and antioxidant roles. Results from the Third National Health and Nutrition Examination Survey, conducted by the Centers for Disease Control and Prevention, found that carotenoids in the diet are inversely associated with fasting serum insulin. Carotenoids are also known to protect the heart. Researchers agree that getting the spectrum of carotenoids is the best strategy to improve your health and get their maximum antioxidant benefits.

 Kitchen Prescription

Fourteen-Carrot Protection! As fat-soluble compounds, you can get the most protection from carotenoid-rich foods such as carrots, butternut squash, and sweet potatoes, to name a few, by cooking them and adding a little oil. It helps make the phytonutrients more available to your body so more get into your bloodstream to boost nutrition.

Lycopene. This powerful antioxidant is well known for its scavenging ability on free radicals. Studies show lycopene protects the heart by reducing the oxidation of LDL cholesterol.

Healing Tip

Love Your Lycopene! Other than tomatoes, you can get lycopene in watermelons, guavas, papaya, apricots, pink grapefruit, and blood oranges. It's fat soluble too, so cook those tomatoes well, add some extra-virgin olive oil, and toss with your favorite pasta!

Organosulfur Compounds

Mainly found in the broccoli (Cruciferae) family of vegetables, organosulfur compounds have potent antioxidant activity and are best known for their ability to fight cancer. In this family of phytonutrients you will find isothiocyanates, indoles, and several others.

Healing Tip

Cellular Defense! Eat your cruciferous veggies for their potent antioxidant action. Get these fabulous phytonutrients in vegetables including broccoli, cauliflower, cabbage, kale, watercress, collards, and radishes.

Allylic Sulfur Compounds

Derived mainly from the allium, or onion, family, these phytonutrients give the characteristic bite to onions, garlic, and other relatives of this bulb group. These compounds have been found to stabilize blood sugar, protect the heart, and fight cancer.

A 2003 study published in the *Journal of Nutrition* examined the effects of garlic powder extracts (either grown with sulfur fertilizer or without) on cytokine levels in blood. The study found that garlic extract reduced cytokines in the blood and in surrounding tissues.

Ajoene is a compound found in garlic and is known for its blood-thinning and cholesterol-lowering properties.

Allicin is a compound formed in garlic when an intact clove of garlic is crushed. An odorless amino acid, allicin is enzymatically converted by allinase into allicin when the cloves are crushed. Allicin is thought to be one of the most biologically active compounds in garlic protecting against LDL cholesterol.

Sulfides are also found in garlic as well as in cabbage, broccoli, brussels sprouts, and other members of the crucifer family. *Diallyl disulfide* (*DADS*), a substance that is formed from the compounds present in garlic, is known to increase levels of detoxifying enzymes in the body, including glutathione.

Kitchen Prescription

A Little Goes a Long Way! Don't let anyone tell you garlic breath isn't beautiful. Crush it and mix in with a simple dressing of extra-virgin olive oil and balsamic vinegar, and drizzle over a big mixed green salad full of phytonutrients or enjoy it in our recipe here for Garlicky Bruschetta.

Garlicky Bruschetta
4 tomatoes, chopped
4 garlic cloves, crushed
½ shallot, diced
½ cup fresh basil, chopped
¼ cup extra-virgin olive oil
8 slices whole-grain Italian bread, sliced

Mix all ingredients together, except for bread. Let stand for 10 minutes. Toast bread and top with tomato mixture for a dose of ajoene, allicin, sulfides, and lycopene.

Serves 8 (serving size: 1 slice bread with ¼ cup tomato mixture)

Now that you have learned about the spectrum of fertility-boosting nutrients, fats, and carbohydrates, the next chapter examines the individual foods that work together—in synergy—to help you take control of your health.

For the Boys: Increasing Vitality Through Diet

As we discussed in Chapter 1, the morphology (shape) and motility (movement) of sperm greatly affect its ability to successfully fertilize an egg. So, too, does the number of sperm (sperm count). Research shows that damage made by free radicals greatly affects the quality of both sperm and eggs, reducing fertility.

Nutrients to Be Fruitful

As discussed in the previous chapter, nutrients have taught us few new things in recent decades. However, only recently have we begun to understand their individual roles in facilitating fertility and preventing disease. Along with the antioxidant-rich "Foods to Be Fruitful" in Chapter 6, here we'll look at some of the specific nutrients found to boost sperm count, benefit the shape and movement of sperm, and the foods you can find them in. We offer information on the vitamins and minerals as a percentage of the daily value (DV) for men fifty and under. Talk with your registered dietitian to meet your personal nutritional needs.

Vitamin B$_{12}$

Vitamin B$_{12}$ has an important role in a process called *methylation* to DNA. This critical process ensures proper division of genetic material, including sperm. A 2003 study found that vitamin B$_{12}$ deficiency reduced the speed of sperm by 20 to 40 percent and increased the number of abnormal sperm. Another recent study found that free radicals have damaging effects to the morphology and motility of sperm; the more vitamin B$_{12}$ and folacin in the semen, the less sperm-squelching free radicals.

 Healing Tip

Go Fish! Vitamin B$_{12}$ is found in clams (84.1 mcg or 1,400 percent DV), trout (5.4 mcg or 90 percent DV), salmon (4.9 mcg or 80 percent DV), yogurt (1.4 mcg or 25 percent DV), tuna (1 mcg or 15 percent DV), and milk (0.9 mcg or 15 percent DV).

Folate

Folate, like vitamin B$_{12}$, plays an important role in DNA division. A 2001 study published in *Fertility Sterility* found that folate levels are correlated significantly with sperm density and total sperm count. A 2002 study published in the same journal showed that folate (5 mg/day) and zinc (66 mg/day) supplementation in men considered "subfertile" increased sperm count by 74 percent.

Healing Tip

Get folate in black-eyed peas (105 mcg or 25 percent DV), cooked spinach (100 mcg or 25 percent DV), great northern beans (90 mcg or 20 percent DV), asparagus (85 mcg or 20 percent DV), wheat germ (40 mcg or 10 percent DV), orange juice (35 mcg or 10 percent DV), peas (50 mcg or 15 percent DV), cooked broccoli (45 mcg or 15 percent DV), avocados (45 mcg or 10 percent DV), and peanuts (40 mcg or 10 percent DV).

Vitamin C

Antioxidants, by way of reducing the damage free radicals cause to DNA and tissues, have been found to benefit sperm count, motility, and morphology. Vitamin C is thought to reduce *DNA fragmentation* or genetic damage to sperm cells known to compromise male fertility. A 2005 study published in *Human Reproduction* found an association between total sperm count and levels of vitamin C.

Healing Tip

Get your daily dose of vitamin C in medium oranges (78 mg or 104 percent DV), medium grapefruit (132 mg or 178 percent DV), blueberries (14 mg or 19 percent DV), strawberries (122 mg or 163 percent DV), mangoes (57 mg or 76 percent), papayas (94 mg or 125 percent DV), cantaloupe (70 mg or 93 percent), watermelons (12 mg or 16 percent DV), sweet potatoes (18 mg or 24 percent DV), green peppers (95 mg or 125 percent DV), and red peppers (226 mg or 301 percent DV).

Vitamin E

As a fat-soluble antioxidant, vitamin E helps to protect DNA from free radical damage. A 2005 study published in *Human Reproduction* found that vitamin E in the diet is associated with both sperm count and motility.

 Kitchen Prescription

Es to Please! Vitamin E is found in wheat germ oil (20.3 mg or 100 percent DV), almonds (7.4 mg or 40 percent DV), sunflower seeds (6 mg or 40 percent DV), hazelnuts (4.3 mg or 20 percent DV), peanuts (2.2 mg or 10 percent DV), mangoes (0.9 mg or 6 percent DV), broccoli (1.2 mg or 6 percent DV), spinach (1.6 mg or 6 percent DV), and kiwis (1.1 mg or 6 percent DV).

Beta-Carotene

Like vitamin E, beta-carotene is a potent fat-soluble antioxidant that helps prevent damage to DNA. A 2005 study evaluated the diets of ninety-seven men using a food-frequency questionnaire. The study found that the men eating more beta-carotene-rich foods had higher sperm concentration and better motility.

 Healing Tip

Get It Whole! Get your beta-carotene in sweet potatoes, carrots, cantaloupe, squash, apricots, pumpkins, and mangoes. Add heat and a little oil for optimum benefits.

Zinc

Zinc is an essential mineral found in almost every cell in the body and is contained within more than two hundred enzymes. It's important for a healthy immune system, for healing, and for maintaining your sense of taste and smell. Zinc also supports normal growth and development during pregnancy, childhood, and adolescence, and studies show that zinc levels are lower in infertile men. A 2002 study published in *Fertility Sterility* showed that folate (5 mg/day) and zinc (66 mg/day) supplementation in men considered "subfertile" increased sperm count by 74 percent!

 Healing Tip

Get zinc in oysters (16 mg or 100 percent DV), ready-to-eat breakfast cereal fortified with zinc (15 mg or 100 percent DV), low-fat yogurt (2.2 mg or 15 percent DV), baked beans (1.7 mg or 10 percent DV), cashews (1.6 mg or 10 percent DV), pecans (1.4 mg or 10 percent DV), chickpeas (1.3 mg or 8 percent DV), almonds (1 mg or 6 percent DV), walnuts (1 mg or 6 percent DV), chicken (1 mg or 6 percent DV), and cheese (1 mg or 6 percent DV).

Selenium

Although selenium is a mineral rather than a nutrient, it is a component of antioxidant enzymes. Selenium helps to protect cells against the effects of free radicals produced during normal metabolism. In animal studies, a selenium deficiency causes immotile, deformed sperm and infertility. Scientists have found that selenium plays an important role with glutathione in producing the correct architecture of sperm for fertility.

Healing Tip

Brazil nuts contain large quantities of selenium (540 mg or 780 percent DV). You can also find it in tuna (63 mg or 95 percent DV), cod (32 mg or 45 percent DV), turkey (32 mg or 45 percent DV), chicken (20 mg or 30 percent DV), noodles (17 mg or 25 percent DV), and oatmeal (12 mg or 15 percent DV).

Glutathione

Glutathione is a cellular antioxidant and detoxifying system. This system helps to prevent free radical damage, as well as maintain the integrity of male and female sex cells—both important to prevent fertility problems. Together with selenium, glutathione helps to develop the architecture of sperm.

 Healing Tip

Feel good about adding glutathione to your antioxidant armory with avocados, asparagus, tomatoes, strawberries, watermelon, and other common foods.

Omega-3 Fats

Omega-3 fatty acids, specifically docosahexaenoic acid (DHA), is a major polyunsaturated fatty acid (PUFA) in human sperm. This PUFA is an important factor in preserving the integrity of DNA and also in how long sperm are motile.

Healing Tip

Get omega-3 fatty acids in flaxseed, walnuts, salmon, tuna, and other cold-water fish. Also look for new food products with enhanced omega-3s, including eggs, breads, frozen waffles, and cereals.

Kitchen Prescriptions

The following recipes are just a few to get you started on your way toward eating better for increased vitality. Be sure to check out Chapter 10 for more delicious recipes filled with foods incorporating these important nutrients for your health.

Father-to-Be Smoothie

Vitamin E, omega-3 fatty acids, vitamin B_{12}, and folate team up to turn up your virility.

½ cup low-fat yogurt
1 cup almond milk
1 tablespoon flaxseed
2 tablespoons wheat germ
½ cup frozen strawberries
½ cup frozen mango

Add all ingredients to a blender. Blend until smooth. Enjoy.

Oysters Delight

Zinc, vitamin E, and folate come together in a dish with age-old aphrodisiac properties. Turn up the heat and turn down the lights!

⅓ cup wheat germ
1 package chopped spinach, cooked with no salt and
     drained
1 tablespoon Parmesan cheese
4 green onion tops, chopped
1 teaspoon Worcestershire sauce
½ teaspoon Tabasco sauce
2 dozen oysters

Mix wheat germ with spinach and Parmesan cheese; add onions, Worcestershire, and Tabasco. Place oysters on a cookie sheet, and top with spinach mixture. Bake at 400°F for 30 minutes.

Nutty Snack Mix

This great snack is a healthy alternative to chips and pretzels, and is filled with nutrient-dense ingredients.

2 cups air-popped popcorn
½ cup raw peanuts
½ cup raw almonds
½ cup raw walnuts
¼ cup raw Brazil nuts
1 teaspoon paprika
1 teaspoon no-salt seasoning mix

Add all ingredients to a large food storage bag. Shake well.

Foods to Be Fruitful

As we've mentioned before, each fruit, vegetable, legume, or grain—like a team player or a note in a symphony—adds a nutritional element valuable to protecting your health, boosting your fertility, and ensuring a healthy pregnancy. Some people are under the dangerous misconception the cost of bad diet can be offset by taking nutritional supplements. *Wrong!* Many phytonutrients have yet to be identified. In addition, other elements, such as fiber, good fats, and the like, aren't in those pills, so you end up fighting the battle against infertility with the wrong weapons. Now that you've learned about the spectrum of nutrients, fats, and carbohydrates, let's look at the individual foods that work together—to increase fertility.

The Synergy of Foods

With the diligent work of scientists worldwide and the evolution of technology, we have isolated and identified approximately 25,000 unique phytonutrients in hundreds of different types of plant foods. Through research, we're learning that by combining these foods, the bioactive compounds work together—or synergistically—to increase health benefits. For example, when oranges, apples, grapes, and blueberries were tested both alone and together, the antioxidant activity was five times lower for the individual fruit than the combined fruit "salad."

Although particular groups of fruits and vegetables have been found to be especially protective for balancing blood sugar—such as legumes—research has pointed to the conclusion that achieving a healthy weight, stabilizing blood sugar, boosting fertility, and preventing disease are best achieved by food synergy. While there are many phytonutrients that act as part of your fertility support team, you don't need to memorize them to get the benefits. Let's explore the families of foods and their unique properties (as seen in Table 6.1).

TABLE 6.1 Foods and Their Fertility-Boosting Properties

Group/Family	Foods	Phytonutrients
Cruciferae (crucifer family)	Broccoli, brussels sprouts, cabbage, cauliflower, collard greens, kale, kohlrabi, mustard greens, radishes, rutabaga, turnips, watercress	Isothiocyanates, indoles, nitriles, sulforaphane, chlorophyll
Cucurbitaceae (the melon and squash family)	Cantaloupes, cucumbers, honeydew melons, summer squash (pumpkin, zucchini), winter squash (acorn, butternut)	Carotenoids, beta-carotene, alpha-carotene, beta-cryptoxanthin, zeaxanthin, lutein
Labitae (mint family)	Basil, mint, oregano, rosemary, sage, thyme	Terpenoids, menthol, chlorophyll

Leguminoseae (bean family)	Alfalfa sprouts, beans, peas, soybeans	Phytoestrogens, lignans, protease inhibitors, isoflavones, saponins
Liliaceae (lily family)	Asparagus, chives, garlic, leeks, onions, shallots	Sulfur compounds, sulfides, allicin, diallyl sulfide
Rutacea (citrus family)	*Grapefruits, lemons, limes, oranges, tangerines	Limonene, carotenoids, lycopene (blood oranges and pink grapefruits), vitamin C
Solanaceae (solanum/ nightshade family)	Eggplant, peppers, potatoes, tomatoes	Lycopene, carotenoids, terpenes
Umbelliferae (umbel family)	Anise, caraway, carrots, celeriac, celery, chervil, cilantro, coriander, cumin, dill, fennel, parsley, parsnips	Carotenoids, beta-carotene, alpha-carotene, beta-cryptoxanthin, zeaxanthin, lutein, chlorophyll
Zingiberaceae (ginger family)	Ginger, turmeric	Curcumin, gingerols, zingibain
Theaceae (tea family)	Black tea, green tea, oolong tea, white tea varieties	Catechins, polyphenols, epigallocatechin gallate (EGCG), theaflavins

* Check with your doctor before eating grapefruit, as it can have interactions with different medications, especially statins (medications that help to lower cholesterol).

Color-Coded Cuisine

Use your plate like a canvas and paint to your heart's content! David Heber, Ph.D., of the UCLA Center for Human Nutrition in Los Angeles introduced a concept that groups foods by color to simplify eating for optimum health and disease prevention. It is not necessary to know the names of the thousands of phytonutrients present in foods to reap their health benefits. In fact, choosing a variety of foods from all of the families we have described offers the complete spectrum of nutrients needed to protect you from disease. The same phytonutrients that keep your cells healthy also give fruits and vegetables their colors and indicate their unique physiological roles. By color coding your cuisine, you can translate the science of phytonutrient nutrition into delicious dishes. The following list more closely examines what the colors mean.

❖ **Blue and purple.** Blue and purple fruits and vegetables contain varying amounts of health-promoting phytonutrients, such as anthocyanins and phenolics. Anthocyanins are currently being studied for their beneficial effects on fat cells and their ability to reduce inflammatory cytokines.

❖ **Green.** Green vegetables contain varying amounts of phytonutrients such as lutein and indoles, which interest researchers because of their potential antioxidant, health-promoting benefits.

❖ **White.** White, tan, and brown fruits and vegetables contain varying amounts of phytonutrients of interest to scientists. These include sulfides and allicin, found in the garlic and onion family, which help stabilize blood sugar, promote a healthy weight, and protect the heart by reducing the oxidation of LDL cholesterol.

❖ **Yellow and orange.** Yellow and orange fruits and vegetables contain varying amounts of antioxidants such as vitamin C as well as carotenoids and flavonoids. Flavonoids are potent antioxidants that can help reduce fertility-wrecking free radicals, while carotenoids play a role in reducing insulin resistance.

❖ **Red.** Lycopene and anthocyanins are the specific phytonutrients in the red group that are being studied for their health-promoting properties. Lycopene, a powerful antioxidant found in the highest concentrations in cooked tomato products, is particularly protective of the heart.

A to Z Foods: Your Fertility-Boosting Team

Balance your blood sugar, achieve a healthy weight, and, ladies, get your body ready for pregnancy—deliciously! In this section, we take the colors one step further and discover the individual foods in the fertility-boosting team. We'll also show you what to look for when selecting, how to store for optimum flavor and nutritional benefits, and some recipes from Chapter 10 that incorporate these foods. Please note that the list in this book is limited, so visit our website at healinggourmet.com for more information.

Apples

Grown in temperate zones throughout the world and cultivated for at least 3,000 years, apple varieties now number well into the thousands. The apple has been called the "king of fruits," and for good reason. The quercetin found in the peel of your apples helps to reduce inflammatory cytokines and protect the insulin-secreting cells of the pancreas. These kingly fruits also provide sugar-balancing soluble fiber called *pectin* that also helps to reduce cholesterol.

❖ **Serving.** One apple (5 oz) with skin contains 81 calories, 0.3 gram protein, 22 grams carbohydrates, no fat, no cholesterol, and 5 grams dietary fiber. The same serving provides 13 percent of the RDA for vitamin C (4.8 mg) and 8 percent of the RDA for vitamin E (0.8 mg).

❖ **Selecting and storing.** Available year-round, apples' peak season is from September through November when newly harvested. Buy firm, well-colored apples with a fresh (never musty) fragrance. The skins should be smooth and free of bruises and gouges. Store apples in a cool, dark place. They do well placed in a plastic bag and stored in the refrigerator.

 Kitchen Prescription

Try our Cabbage and Apple Slaw for a fiber and quercetin-rich accompaniment to any meal.

Apricots

Born in China some 4,000 years ago, apricots are widely consumed by the long-living Hunza people. The cousin of the peach arrived in California with the Spanish in the eighteenth century.

❖ **Serving.** Three apricots (4 oz) contains 51 calories, 1.5 grams protein, 11.8 grams carbohydrates, 0.5 gram fat, no cholesterol, and 2 grams dietary fiber. The same serving provides 28 percent of the RDA for vitamin A (200 RE), 14 percent of the RDA for vitamin C (10.5 mg), 2 percent of the RDA for iron (0.4 mg), and 272 milligrams of potassium. The apricot also contains salicylates, boron, and carotenoids.

❖ **Selecting and storing.** Because they're highly perishable and seasonal, 90 percent of the fresh apricots are marketed in June and July. When buying apricots, select plump, reasonably firm fruit with a uniform color. Store in a plastic bag in the refrigerator for three to five days. Depending on size, there are eight to twelve apricots per pound.

Healing Tip

The yellow color of these little beauties is due to carotenoids that have been found to have an inverse relation to fasting serum insulin in the Third National Health and Nutrition Examination Survey conducted by the Centers for Disease Control and Prevention.

Artichokes

Vegetable flowers that are picked and eaten before they turn into a "real" flower, artichokes are a European staple. These gorgeous globes provide a good amount of fiber and folate.

❖ **Serving.** One artichoke, boiled (4.2 oz) contains 60 calories, 4.2 grams protein, 13.4 grams carbohydrates, 0.2 gram fat, no cholesterol, and 6.5 grams dietary fiber. The same serving provides 15 percent of the RDA for folate (61.2 mcg), 16 percent of the RDA for vitamin C (12 mg), 12 percent of the RDA for magnesium (47 mg), 11 percent of the RDA for iron (1.6 mg), and 316 milligrams of potassium. Artichokes also contain cynaroside, luteolin, dicaffeoylquinic and dicaffeoyltartaric acids.

❖ **Selecting and storing.** Globe artichokes are available year-round, with the peak season from March through May. Buy deep green, heavy-for-their-size artichokes with a tight leaf formation. The leaves should "squeak" when pressed together. Heavy browning on an artichoke usually indicates it's beyond its prime. Store unwashed artichokes in a plastic bag in the refrigerator for up to four days; wash just before cooking. Artichoke hearts are available frozen and canned; artichoke bottoms are available canned.

Kitchen Prescription

Canned artichoke hearts are a delicious addition to salads, chicken dishes, and pasta. Just drain and toss into your favorite dish for a nutritional boost.

Asparagus

A member of the lily family, the edible part of asparagus is actually the young underground sprout or shoot. Asparagus provides glutathione, an antioxidant compound that may help to keep blood sugar stable and regulate blood pressure, and almost half of the recommended daily intake for folate.

❖ **Serving.** One-half cup of raw asparagus contains 15 calories, 1.5 grams protein, 2.5 grams carbohydrates, 0.1 gram fat, no cholesterol, and 1.3 grams dietary fiber. The same serving provides 6 percent of the RDA for vitamin A (60 RE), 48 percent of the RDA for folate (95 mcg), 37 percent of the RDA for vitamin C (22.1 mg), 5 percent of the RDA for vitamin B_6 (0.1 mg), 3 percent of the RDA for iron (0.4 mg), and 218 milligrams of potassium.

❖ **Selecting and storing.** The optimum season for fresh asparagus lasts from February through June, although hothouse asparagus is available year-round in some regions. It's best cooked the same day it's purchased but will keep, tightly wrapped in a plastic bag, three to four days in the refrigerator. Or, store standing upright in about an inch of water, covering the container with a plastic bag.

Kitchen Prescription

Get these spears of protection in our Asparagus, Mushroom, and Tomato Melt.

Avocados

Native to the tropics and subtropics, avocados are a unique fruit and concentrated source of nutrients. The California avocado has a smooth skin, while the Florida avocado (or alligator pear) has a tough and wrinkled exterior. More like a nut than a fruit, these South American natives supply heart-healthy monounsaturated fat and vitamin B_6, magnesium to bolster insulin function, and glutathione for antioxidant protection. Holy guacamole!

✤ **Serving.** One (6 oz) avocado contains 204 calories, 3.8 grams protein, 13.3 grams carbohydrates, 17 grams fat, no cholesterol, and 9.3 grams dietary fiber. The same serving provides 19 percent of the RDA for vitamin A (186 RE), 15 percent of the RDA for folate (60 mcg), 40 percent of the RDA for vitamin C (24 mg), 8 percent of the RDA for vitamin B_6 (0.13 mg), 30 percent of the RDA for niacin (5.9 mg), 27 percent of the RDA for thiamin (0.4 mg), 26 percent of the RDA for magnesium (104 mg), 22 percent of the RDA for riboflavin (0.4 mg), 11 percent of the RDA for iron (1.6 mg), and 1,484 milligrams of potassium.

✤ **Selecting and storing.** Like many fruits, avocados ripen best off the tree. Ripe avocados yield to gentle palm pressure, but firm, unripe avocados are what are usually found in the market. Select those that are unblemished and heavy for their size. To speed the ripening process, place several avocados in a paper bag and set aside at room temperature for two to four days. Ripe avocados can be stored in the refrigerator several days. Once avocado flesh is cut and exposed to the air it tends to discolor rapidly; adding lemon or lime juice helps to prevent discoloration.

 Kitchen Prescription

Guacamole is a snap to make and adds flavor and nutrients to sandwiches, wraps, and whole-grain crackers. Chop 1 large avocado, add 1 teaspoon paprika, 2 tablespoons lemon juice, and ½ cup diced onion. Mash together and enjoy!

Barley

Beige and shaped like a flattened oval, this grain is usually sold pearled, where it is hulled and polished to cook more quickly. Hulled (also called *whole-grain*) barley has only the outer husk removed and is the most nutritious form of the grain. Scotch barley is husked and coarsely ground. Pearl barley has also had the bran removed and has been steamed and polished. It comes in three sizes: coarse, medium, and fine and is good in soups and stews. Barley can also be found in quick-cooking, whole-hulled, Job's tears (large-hulled grains) grits flakes, and flour varieties. Used to make beer, whiskey, and cattle feed, barley is a gluten grain that should be avoided by those with gluten sensitivity. Barley helps to balance blood sugar and fight free radicals with its tocotrienols (a form of vitamin E).

✦ **Serving.** One-half cup of pearled barley contains 97 calories, 1.8 grams protein, 22.3 grams carbohydrates, 0.4 gram fat, no cholesterol, and 4.4 grams dietary fiber. The same serving provides 6 percent of the RDA for folate (12.6 mcg), 8 percent of the RDA for niacin (1.6 mg), and 7 percent of the RDA for iron (1.1 mg).

✤ **Selecting and storing.** Barley grits are hulled barley grains that have been cracked into medium-coarse pieces. Hulled and Scotch barley and barley grits are generally found in health-food stores. Store in an airtight container in a cool, dry place.

 Healing Tip

Opt for hulled barley that still has its germ and bran layers intact, to help keep blood sugar on an even keel.

Beans

Part of the legume family, a good protein source, and a low-GI food, beans provide a bevy of phytonutrients to boost fertility, promote a healthy weight, and protect the heart. Filled with phytoestrogens, insoluble fiber, calcium, and folate, these packages of protection are a mainstay in your diet for optimum health.

✤ **Serving.** One-half cup of cooked black beans contains 113 calories, 7.6 grams protein, 20.4 grams carbohydrates, 0.4 gram fat, no cholesterol, and 7.5 grams dietary fiber. The same serving size provides 32 percent of the RDA for folate (64.2 mcg), 13 percent of the RDA for magnesium (51.6 mg), and 270.2 milligrams of potassium.

✤ **Selecting and storing.** Dried beans must usually be soaked in water for several hours or overnight to rehydrate them before cooking. Beans labeled "quick-cooking" have been presoaked and redried before packaging; they require no presoaking and take considerably less time to prepare. The texture of these "quick" beans, however, is not as firm to the bite as regular dried beans. Store dried beans in an airtight container for up to a year.

Kitchen Prescription

Try our Pea in the Pod Soup to ladle on the protection.

Blueberries

These berries have been enjoyed by Native Americans and pilgrims and are one of the best-known sources of antioxidants. A true-blue health crusader, blueberries provide anthocyanins that have beneficial effects on fat cells and help to reduce inflammatory cytokines.

✢ **Serving.** One cup of blueberries contains 82 calories, 1 gram protein, 20.5 grams carbohydrates, 0.6 gram fat, no cholesterol, and 3.5 grams dietary fiber. The same serving provides 315 percent of the RDA for vitamin C (189 mg) and 129 milligrams of potassium.

✢ **Selecting and storing.** Choose blueberries that are firm, uniform in size, and indigo blue with a silvery frost. Discard shriveled or moldy berries. Do not wash until ready to use, and store (preferably in a single layer) in a moisture-proof container in the refrigerator for up to five days.

 Kitchen Prescription

Get these blue gems in our Mixed Berry Scones. Or, buy them frozen, microwave, and add to breakfast cereal for a no-fuss fix full of flavor and phytonutrients.

Broccoli

A descendant of cabbage, broccoli is a member of the cruciferous family of vegetables. Although most broccoli is green, in past times, purple, red, cream, and brown varieties were popular. Broccoli contains quercetin—a flavonoid found to help reduce inflammatory cytokines and protect our insulin-secreting cells—plus baby-boosting folate, vitamin C, and vitamin B_6.

❖ **Serving.** One-half cup of cooked broccoli contains 23 calories, 2.3 grams protein, 6 grams carbohydrates, 0.2 gram fat, no cholesterol, and 2.6 grams dietary fiber. The same serving provides 11 percent of the RDA for vitamin A (110 RE), 27 percent of the RDA for folate (53.3 mcg), 82 percent of the RDA for vitamin C (49 mg), 10 percent of the RDA for vitamin B_6 (0.2 mg), 6 percent of the RDA for iron (0.9 mg), and 127 milligrams of potassium.

❖ **Selecting and storing.** Look for broccoli with a deep, strong color—green or green with purple. The buds should be tightly closed and the leaves should be crisp. Refrigerate unwashed, in an airtight bag, for up to four days.

 Kitchen Prescription

Get broccoli in our Garden Garbanzo Soup. Or lightly steam broccoli, and add a squeeze of lemon and a shake of Parmesan cheese for the perfect accompaniment to virtually any meal.

Buckwheat

A triangular seed from a fruit relative of rhubarb and sorrel, buckwheat has a nutty flavor and is sold roasted (kasha), whole-grain cracked, unroasted groats grits, or ground into flour. A whole grain and good source of phytonutrients, buckwheat may help to stabilize blood sugar and reduce inflammation.

✤ **Serving.** One-half cup of buckwheat groats (cooked) contains 77 calories, 2.8 grams protein, 16.8 grams carbohydrate, 0.5 gram fat, no cholesterol, and no dietary fiber. The same serving provides 7 percent of the RDA for folate (13.9 mcg), 13 percent of the RDA for magnesium (43 mg), and 5 percent of the RDA for iron (0.8 mg).

✤ **Selecting and storing.** Buckwheat groats are the hulled, crushed kernels, which are usually cooked in a manner similar to rice. Groats come in coarse, medium, and fine grinds. Kasha, which is roasted buckwheat groats, has a toastier, more nutty flavor. All can be stored in an airtight container in a cool, dry place.

 Healing Tip

For more information on how whole grains, such as buckwheat, help to stabilize blood sugar and promote fertility, refer back to Chapter 3.

Canola Oil

Derived from canola seed and produced in Canada, this oil contains the lowest level of saturated fat of any other oil. Canola oil provides fertility-friendly fat—including omega-3 fatty acids—which have been found to reduce inflammation, increase the flow of blood to the uterus, and boost your child's brainpower.

✤ **Serving.** One tablespoon contains 124 calories, no protein, no carbohydrates, 14 grams fat, 1 gram saturated fatty acids, 8 grams monounsaturated fatty acids, 4.2 grams polyunsaturated fatty acids, 1.2 grams omega-3s, no cholesterol, and no dietary fiber. The same serving provides 13 percent of the RDA for vitamin E (2.9 mg).

✤ **Selecting and storing.** Store canola oil in a cool, dry place away from sunlight.

 Kitchen Prescription

This light oil is perfect for sautéing, using in baked goods, or spraying to reduce food from sticking on a grill or skillet.

Cantaloupes

This orange-fleshed melon was named after the Italian town of Cantalupa, which also means "wolf howl." The orange color of this juicy melon provides a powerful punch of carotenoids that act as antioxidants and may benefit insulin function, plus vitamin C, folate, and vitamin B_6.

✤ **Serving.** One-half raw cantaloupe (9.5 oz) contains 95 calories, 2.5 grams protein, 22.4 grams carbohydrates, 0.8 gram fat, no cholesterol, and 2.5 grams dietary fiber. The same serving provides 86 percent of the RDA for vitamin A (861 RE), 23 percent of the RDA for folate (45.5 mcg), 186 percent of the RDA for vitamin C (112.7 mg), 20 percent of the RDA for vitamin B_6 (0.4 mg), and 825 milligrams of potassium.

✤ **Selecting and storing.** Choose cantaloupes that are heavy for their size; have a sweet, fruity fragrance and a thick, well-raised netting; and yield slightly to pressure at the blossom end. Avoid melons with soft spots or an overly strong odor. Store unripe cantaloupes at room temperature and ripe melons in the refrigerator. Cantaloupes easily absorb other food odors so if refrigerating for more than a day or two, wrap the melon in plastic wrap.

Healing Tip

Before cutting into these delicious melons, make sure you wash well, as bacteria from the outside gets transferred to the inside with the knife blade. Find out more about the dangers of food contamination and pregnancy in Chapter 7.

Carrots

As root vegetables that spread from the Middle East to Greece, Rome, and later to Europe, the earliest carrots were not orange, but multicolored. In the 1500s, the carrot showed up in Western Europe, and Dutch cross-breeders developed the modern, orange carrot over the following century. Of course, carrots are full of carotenoids—those antioxidant compounds that help keep insulin in check and protect the heart.

✤ **Serving.** One medium carrot (2.5 oz) contains 31 calories, 0.7 gram protein, 5.6 grams carbohydrates, 0.1 gram fat, no cholesterol, and 2 grams dietary fiber. The same serving also provides 202 percent of the RDA for vitamin A (2,025 RE), 5 percent of the RDA for folate (10 mcg), 11 percent of the RDA for vitamin C (6.7 mg), and 233 milligrams of potassium.

✤ **Selecting and storing.** When selecting carrots, choose ones that are firm and smooth. Avoid those with cracks or any that have begun to soften and wither. Remove carrot greenery as soon as possible because it robs the roots of moisture and vitamins. Store carrots in a plastic bag in the refrigerator's vegetable bin. Avoid storing them near apples, which emit ethylene gas that can give carrots a bitter taste.

Kitchen Prescription

Get Bugs Bunny's favorite food in our Moroccan Fish Tagine.

Cherries

Close cousins to the plum, cherries can be sweet or sour, or red or black. Pick cherries for their abundance of antioxidant flavonoids and anthocyanins that help to reduce the inflammatory cytokines that contribute to insulin resistance and PCOS.

❖ **Serving.** Ten sweet, raw cherries (2.4 oz) contain 50 calories, 0.9 gram protein, 11.3 grams carbohydrates, 0.7 gram fat, no cholesterol, and 1.5 grams dietary fiber. The same serving provides 8 percent of the RDA for vitamin C (4.8 mg), 2 percent of the RDA for iron (0.3 mg), and 152 milligrams of potassium.

❖ **Selecting and storing.** Most fresh cherries are available from May (June for sour cherries) through August. Choose brightly colored, shiny, plump cherries. Sweet cherries should be firm, but not hard; sour varieties should be medium-firm. Store unwashed cherries in a plastic bag in the refrigerator.

 Kitchen Prescription

Not the Pits! Buy cherries frozen, then microwave and add to yogurts or breakfast cereals for health on high speed.

Cranberries

Grown in bogs throughout Asia, Europe, and North America, these berries are best known for a Thanksgiving celebration and their ability to reduce the incidence of bladder infections. These tart treats contain inflammation-reducing anthocyanins. Cranberries also contain oxalic acid.

❖ **Serving.** One cup of raw cranberries contains 46 calories, 0.4 gram protein, 12.1 grams carbohydrates, 0.2 gram fat, no cholesterol, and 4.4 grams dietary fiber. The same serving provides 21 percent of the RDA for vitamin C (12.8 mg).

❖ **Selecting and storing.** Harvested between Labor Day and Halloween, the peak market period for cranberries is from October through December. They're usually packaged in twelve-ounce plastic bags. Any cranberries that are discolored or shriveled should be discarded. Cranberries can be refrigerated, tightly wrapped, for up to two months or frozen up to a year.

 Kitchen Prescription

Try our whole-grain Cranberry Walnut Squares for a delicious breakfast or light dessert with benefits.

Eggplants

A flowering vegetable native to India, the many varieties of this delicious veggie range in color from rich purple to white, in length from two to twelve inches, and in shape from oblong to round. With purple anthocyanins to reduce inflammation, this giant berry makes a healthy and hearty alternative to meat dishes.

❖ **Serving.** One-half cup of cooked eggplant contains 13 calories, 0.4 gram protein, 3.2 grams carbohydrates, 0.1 gram fat, no cholesterol, and 1.2 grams dietary fiber. The same serving provides 3 percent of the RDA for folate (6.9 mcg) and 119 milligrams of potassium.

❖ **Selecting and storing.** Available year-round, eggplant's peak season is August and September. Choose a firm, smooth-skinned eggplant heavy for its size; avoid ones with soft or brown spots. They should be stored in a cool, dry place and used within a day or two of purchase. If longer storage is necessary, place the eggplant in the refrigerator vegetable drawer.

 Kitchen Prescription

Try our Summer Ratatouille for a meatless meal full of fiber and protein.

Flaxseed

Flaxseed was an ancient culinary staple used as early as 3000 B.C. and touted for its ability to relieve intestinal discomfort by Hippocrates. It has a mild, nutty flavor and is often used simply sprinkled over hot dishes such as cooked cereal or stir-fries. This tiny seed provides essential omega-3 fatty acids to help stabilize blood sugar and promote fertility. It is best to consume flax in the ground form because the whole seeds are difficult for our bodies to digest, and therefore you won't reap all of its health benefits.

❖ **Serving.** Two tablespoons of ground flaxseed contains 80 calories, 3.2 grams protein, no carbohydrates, 5.5 grams fat, no cholesterol, and 4.5 grams dietary fiber.

❖ **Selecting and storing.** Store in the refrigerator or freezer, where it will keep for up to six months.

Kitchen Prescription

The omega-3s are also beneficial for sperm production and motility, so try our Carrot Flax Muffins and have a delicious breakfast in bed with your partner.

Garlic

A member of the allium, or onion family, three major types of garlic are available in the United States: the white-skinned, strongly flavored American garlic; the Mexican garlic; and the Italian garlic. The Mexican and Italian varieties both have mauve-colored skins and a somewhat milder flavor. Elephant garlic (which is not a true garlic but a relative of the leek) is the most mild flavored of the three. Garlic delivers blood-sugar balancing and inflammation-reducing phytonutrients including quercetin, allicin, and sulfides.

❖ **Serving.** One ounce of garlic contains no calories, no protein, no carbohydrates, no fat, no cholesterol, and no dietary fiber. The same serving provides 15 percent of vitamin C and vitamin B_6.

❖ **Selecting and storing.** Fresh garlic is available year-round. Purchase firm, plump bulbs with dry skins. Avoid heads with soft or shriveled cloves and those stored in the refrigerated section of the produce department. Store fresh garlic in an open container (away from other foods) in a cool, dark place. Properly stored, unbroken bulbs can be kept for up to eight weeks, though they will begin to dry out toward the end of that time. Once broken from the bulb, individual cloves will keep from three to ten days.

Kitchen Prescription

Get these cloves of protection in our Maternity Minestrone.

Ginger

A member of the Zingiberaceae family that also includes turmeric, most ginger comes from Jamaica, followed by India, Africa, and China. Compounds in ginger called gingerols have been found to improve insulin sensitivity and ginger is an age-old remedy for nausea.

✤ **Serving.** One tablespoon contains 4 calories, 0.1 gram protein, 0.9 gram carbohydrates, 0.1 gram fat, no cholesterol, and 0.1 gram dietary fiber. One tablespoon also provides 46 milligrams of potassium.

✤ **Selecting and storing.** Look for ginger with smooth skin and a fresh, spicy fragrance. Fresh unpeeled gingerroot, tightly wrapped, can be refrigerated for up to three weeks and frozen for up to six months.

Kitchen Prescription

Get your ginger in our Creamy Butternut Squash Soup.

Grapefruit

A member of the citrus family of fruits grown in Florida, the grapefruit has been purported as a weight-loss aid. Providing heart-helping flavonoids and cholesterol-lowering pectin, grapefruit falls on the low end of the glycemic index scale—making it a great choice to control weight and blood sugar levels.

❖ **Serving.** One-half grapefruit contains approximately 45 calories, 1 gram protein, 12 grams carbohydrates, 0.1 gram fat, no cholesterol, and 1.6 grams dietary fiber. The same serving provides 6 percent of the RDA for folate (11.8 mcg) and 66 percent of the RDA for vitamin C (39.3 mg).

❖ **Selecting and storing.** Fresh grapefruit is available year-round. Those from Arizona and California are in the market from about January through August; Florida and Texas grapefruit usually arrive around October and last through June. Choose grapefruit that have thin, fine-textured, brightly colored skin. They should be firm yet springy when held in the palm and pressed. Grapefruit keep best when wrapped in a plastic bag and placed in the vegetable drawer of the refrigerator for up to two weeks.

 Kitchen Prescription

Get a nice helping of grapefruit in our Citrus Refresher. However, grapefruit has numerous interactions with different medications (especially statins), so contact your doctor or pharmacist before consuming grapefruit if you take prescription medication.

Lemons

Citrus fruits cultivated in tropical and temperate climates around the world, lemons add zest and an abundance of vitamin C to foods and beverages. Lemons provide an abundance of free radical–fighting vitamin C and fall low on the glycemic index.

❖ **Serving.** One tablespoon of lemon juice contains 4 calories, 0.1 gram protein, 1.4 grams carbohydrates, no fat, no cholesterol, and no fiber. The same serving provides 11 percent of the RDA for vitamin C (75 mg).

❖ **Selecting and storing.** Lemons are available year-round, peaking during the summer months. Choose fruit with smooth, brightly colored skin with no tinge of green. Lemons should be firm, plump, and heavy for their size. Depending on their condition when purchased, they can be refrigerated in a plastic bag for two to three weeks.

 Kitchen Prescription

Have a "Boca Cocktail," a favorite refreshment of the Boca Raton, Florida, crowd to hydrate you through the day and deliver health-promoting phytonutrients. Just squeeze some fresh lemon into your spring water and voilà!

Lentils

Members of the legume family, lentils come in red, green, and brown varieties. Phytoestrogens and fiber team up to make these high-protein morsels perfect for reducing blood sugar and achieving a healthy weight.

❖ **Serving.** One-half cup cooked contains 101 calories, 7.4 grams protein, 18.4 grams carbohydrates, no fat, no cholesterol, and 9 grams of dietary fiber. The same serving provides 86 percent of the RDA for folate (172.7 mcg), 15 percent of the RDA for iron (0.8 mg), and 7 percent of the RDA for thiamin (0.1 mg).

❖ **Selecting and storing.** Lentils should be stored in an airtight container at room temperature and will keep up to a year.

Kitchen Prescription

Love Your Legumes! Try our Sautéed Cod with Lentils to fill you up without weighing you down!

Mangoes

Cultivated in India for several thousand years, mangoes come in hundreds of varieties. These tropical fruits are high in antioxidants including vitamins C and E, plus carotenoids to help keep insulin in check.

❖ **Serving.** One raw mango contains 128 calories, 1 gram protein, 33.4 grams carbohydrates, 0.6 gram fat, no cholesterol, and 3.7 grams dietary fiber. The same serving provides 77 percent of the RDA for vitamin A (766 RE), 90 percent of the RDA for vitamin C (54 mg), 24 percent of the RDA for vitamin E (2.4 mg), and 14 percent of the RDA for vitamin B_6 (0.28 mg).

❖ **Selecting and storing.** Mangoes are in season from May to September, though imported fruit is in the stores sporadically throughout the remainder of the year. Look for fruit with an unblemished, yellow skin blushed with red.

Kitchen Prescription

Try a unique twist on this tropical delight with our Rice, Bean, and Mango Salad.

Nuts

Scientists speculate nuts may have been around tens of millions of years ago when the continents were still fused—a landmass known as Pangea. We know this because nuts are native to both the Old and New Worlds. Cultivated for twelve thousand years, nuts are one of nature's richest foods. More than three hundred types of nuts exist, but those most commonly enjoyed include almonds, Brazil nuts, cashews, chestnuts, coconuts, hazelnuts, peanuts, pecans, pistachios, walnuts, as well as hickory nuts, pine nuts, and macadamia nuts. Full of protein and minerals and packed with healthy fats, nuts help balance blood sugar and increase fertility.

❖ **Serving.** See individual packages of nuts for serving information.

❖ **Selecting and storing.** Store nuts in closed containers in the refrigerator or freezer to avoid rancidity. It is best to buy fresh raw nuts with shells, as they will store longer than shelled, cooked varieties.

 Kitchen Prescription

Loaded with the "good" fats and minerals, nuts are a great snack and easily incorporated into salads and smoothies. Try our Swiss Muesli for a nutty mix including cashews.

Oats

A highly rich, protein grain eaten in prepared cereals or as a hot cereal, oats are an American staple. The FDA awarded the first food-specific health claim to oats in January 1997 because of their ability to reduce total and LDL cholesterol. Oats also contain tocotrienol, selenium, beta-glucan, and phytates to help keep blood sugar on an even keel.

❖ **Serving.** One cup of cooked oatmeal (½ cup dry) contains 150 calories, 5.5 grams protein, 27 grams carbohydrates, 3 grams fat, no cholesterol, and 4 grams of dietary fiber. The same serving size provides 13 percent of the RDA for thiamin (0.2 mg), 11 percent of the RDA for magnesium (107 mg), and 8 percent of the RDA for iron (1.9 mg).

❖ **Selecting and storing.** Store oats in a cool, dry place and choose steel-cut oats, as they are the most nutritious and least processed.

 Kitchen Prescription

Get these heart-healthy grains in our Cranberry Walnut Squares.

Olive Oil

Most olive oils come from California and are also imported from France, Greece, Italy, and Spain. It is made by pressing tree-ripened olives to extract a flavorful, heart-healthy monounsaturated oil that is prized throughout the world both for cooking and for salads. The flavor, color, and fragrance of olive oils can vary depending on distinctions such as growing region and the crop's condition. Olive oil is also rich in phenolic compounds and oleic acid, which benefit the heart. All olive oils are graded in accordance with the degree of acidity they contain. The best are cold-pressed, a chemical-free process that involves only pressure, which produces a natural level of low acidity. Extra-virgin olive oil, the cold-pressed result of the first pressing of the olives, is only 1 percent acid. It is considered the finest and fruitiest of the olive oils and is therefore also the most expensive. It can range from a champagne color to greenish golden to bright green.

❖ **Serving.** One tablespoon of extra-virgin olive oil contains 120 calories, no protein, no carbohydrates, 14 grams of fat, no cholesterol, and no fiber.

❖ **Selecting and storing.** Olive oil should be stored in a cool, dark place for up to six months. It can be refrigerated, in which case it will last up to a year.

 Healing Tip

In general, the deeper the color, the more intense the olive flavor and more phytonutrients present.

Onions

Members of the allium family, onions have two main classifications: green and dry. Dry onions are simply mature onions with a juicy flesh covered with dry, papery skin. With their inflammation-reducing and blood sugar–balancing sulfur compounds and quercetin, onions add flavor and health to any dish.

❖ **Serving.** One medium, raw onion contains 60 calories, 2 grams protein, 14 grams carbohydrates, no fat, no cholesterol, and 3 grams dietary fiber. The same serving also provides 18 percent of the RDA for vitamin C (12 mg).

❖ **Selecting and storing.** When buying onions, choose ones that are heavy for their size with dry, papery skins and no signs of spotting or moistness. Avoid onions with soft spots. Store in a cool, dry place with good air circulation for up to two months (depending on their condition when purchased). Once cut, an onion should be tightly wrapped, refrigerated, and used within four days.

Kitchen Prescription

Toss them into salads, dice and sauté into sauces, or chop and add to soups. Experiment with different varieties of onions such as cippolini, Texas onions, Vidalia onions, and shallots.

Oranges

The most popular citrus fruit, oranges are believed to have originated in Southeast Asia and were brought to the New World by Christopher Columbus. A low-GI food, oranges also provide flavonoids, carotenoids, glutathione, and folate, which help to reduce inflammation and boost fertility.

✤ **Serving.** One orange (approximately 4.6 oz) contains 62 calories, 1.3 grams protein, 15.4 grams carbohydrates, 0.2 gram fat, no cholesterol, and 3 grams dietary fiber. The same serving provides 20 percent of the RDA for folate (39.7 mcg), 92 percent of the RDA for vitamin C (69.7 mg), 13 percent of the RDA for thiamin (0.2 mg), 4 percent of the RDA for calcium (52 mg), and 237 milligrams of potassium.

✤ **Selecting and storing.** Fresh oranges are available year-round at different times, depending on the variety. Choose fruit that is firm and heavy for its size, with no mold or spongy spots. Oranges can be stored at cool room temperature for a day or so, but should then be refrigerated and kept there for up to two weeks.

Kitchen Prescription

Brighten your day and your health with an orange-juice-based smoothie. Add 1 cup orange juice, 1 cup frozen fruit of your choice, and 1 tablespoon of flaxmeal to a blender. Give it a whirl and enjoy!

Peaches

Widely planted across the eastern seaboard by the early settlers, the peach is the third most popular of all fruits grown in the United States. With their flavonoids, carotenoids, and vitamin C, peaches protect against free radicals and help to keep blood sugar on an even keel.

✤ **Serving.** One peach (approximately 4 oz) contains 37 calories, 0.7 gram protein, 9.7 grams carbohydrates, 0.1 gram fat, no cholesterol, and 1.5 grams dietary fiber. The same serving also provides 47 percent of the RDA for vitamin A (465 RE), 19 percent of the RDA for vitamin C (1.7 mg), and 8 percent of the RDA for niacin (1.5 mg).

✤ **Selecting and storing.** Peaches are available from May to October in most regions of the United States. Look for fragrant fruit that gives slightly to palm pressure. Avoid those with signs of greening.

 Healing Tip

Peaches come in numerous varieties, so enjoy these fuzzy fruits right off the tree for a powerful phytonutrient punch.

Peppers

Thought by the Europeans in the 1600s to cure digestive problems and ulcers, modern medicine has shown that peppers contain numerous compounds that have beneficial effects on the digestive system. Many varieties of peppers exist, including banana peppers, red bell, yellow bell, green bell, chili, cayenne, jalapeno, habanero, and Scotch bonnet. Along with vitamin C, folate, and magnesium, red peppers also give you a dose of lycopene.

✤ **Serving.** One-half of cup red bell pepper contains 14 calories, 0.5 gram protein, 3.2 grams carbohydrates, 0.1 gram fat, no cholesterol, and 1.8 grams dietary fiber. The same serving also provides 11 percent of the RDA for folate (22.2 mcg), 44 percent of the RDA for vitamin C (26.1 mg), 35 percent of the RDA for vitamin B_6 (0.7 mg), 17 percent of the RDA for niacin (3.3 mg), 18 percent of the RDA for thiamin (0.2 mg), 14 percent of the RDA for magnesium (54.5 mg), 19 percent of the RDA for iron (2.8 mg), and 844 milligrams of potassium.

✤ **Selecting and storing.** Choose peppers that are firm; have a brightly colored, shiny skin; and are heavy for their size. Avoid those that are limp, shriveled, or have soft or bruised spots. Store peppers in a plastic bag in the refrigerator for up to a week.

 Kitchen Prescription

Pick a peck of this terrific food in our Stuffed Bell Peppers.

Pomegranates

Unusual fruits with bright red juice and many seeds, the name pomegranate comes from two French words, *pome* and *granate,* which literally means "apple with many seeds." These unique fruits provide a good dose of fiber plus anthocyanins to help reduce inflammatory cytokines.

❖ **Serving.** One pomegranate (approximately 5.5 oz) contains 104 calories, 1.5 grams protein, 26.5 grams carbohydrates, 0.5 gram fat, no cholesterol, and 1 gram dietary fiber. The same serving also provides 16 percent of the RDA for vitamin C (9.4 mg) and 399 milligrams of potassium.

❖ **Selecting and storing.** In the United States they're available in October and November. Choose those that are heavy for their size and have a bright, fresh color and blemish-free skin. Refrigerate for up to two months or store in a cool, dark place.

 Healing Tip

Sprinkle pomegranate buds onto a salad or on top of your favorite cereal in the morning for a delicious dose of anthocyanins.

Pumpkin

A flowering vegetable and members of the gourd family, pumpkins are powerhouses of carotenoids to be enjoyed year-round.

❖ **Serving.** One-half cup of canned pumpkin contains 41 calories, 1.3 grams protein, 9.9 grams carbohydrates, 0.3 gram fat, no cholesterol, and 3.6 grams dietary fiber. The same serving also provides 269 percent of the RDA for vitamin A (2,691 RE), 8 percent of the RDA for folate (15 mcg), 9 percent of the RDA for vitamin C (5.1 mg), 7 percent of the RDA for magnesium (28 mg), 11 percent of the RDA for iron (1.7 mg), and 251 milligrams of potassium.

❖ **Selecting and storing.** Fresh pumpkins are available in the fall and winter, and some specimens have weighed in at well over one hundred pounds. In general, however, the flesh from smaller sizes will be more tender and succulent. Choose pumpkins that are free from blemishes and heavy for their size. Store whole pumpkins at room temperature up to a month or refrigerate up to three months.

 Healing Tip

Buy canned pumpkin year-round and add it to smoothies, breads, muffins, and pancakes.

Raspberries

Typically red, raspberries also come in other colors such as purple, yellow, amber, and black. These antioxidant-rich berries provide flavonoids, folate, and vitamin C.

❖ **Serving.** One cup of raspberries contains 61 calories, 1.2 grams protein, 14.3 grams carbohydrates, 0.7 gram fat, no cholesterol, and 8 grams dietary fiber. The same serving also provides 16 percent of the RDA for folate (32 mcg), 51 percent of the RDA for vitamin C (30.8 mg), 6 percent of the RDA for magnesium (22 mg), and 5 percent of the RDA for iron (0.7 mg).

❖ **Selecting and storing.** Raspberries are available from May through November. Choose brightly colored, plump berries without the hull. If the hulls are still attached, the berries were picked too early and will undoubtedly be tart. Avoid soft, shriveled, or moldy berries. Store in a dry container in the refrigerator for two to three days. If necessary, rinse lightly just before serving.

 Kitchen Prescription

Give our Almond Berry Smoothie a try for a taste temptation full of fertility-boosting nutrients.

Rice

Originating from Southeast Asia, rice is the second most consumed food in the world. Enjoy whole-grain rice with its B vitamins, including B_6, which helps to reduce levels of heart-harming homocysteine, as well as magnesium and thiamin, important for insulin function.

✤ **Serving.** One-half cup of brown rice contains 110 calories, 2.3 grams protein, 23 grams carbohydrates, 0.8 gram fat, no cholesterol, and 1.7 grams dietary fiber. The same serving provides 10 percent of the RDA for vitamin B_6 (0.2 mg), 67 percent of the RDA for thiamin (1 mg), 5 percent of the RDA for niacin (1 mg), 11 percent of the RDA for magnesium (43 mg), and 3 percent of the RDA for iron (0.5 mg).

✤ **Selecting and storing.** Because of the presence of the bran, brown rice is subject to rancidity, which limits its shelf life to only about six months.

 Healing Tip

Don't forget to keep those germ and bran layers on! Buy unrefined brown rice to keep your blood sugar on an even keel.

Soybeans

Members of the legume family and a complete protein, soybeans are a main staple of the Asian diet. Soybeans provide phyto-estrogens, to keep blood sugar in check, and iron, which is impor-tant for a healthy pregnancy.

✤ **Serving.** One-quarter block of tofu (approximately 4 oz) contains 90 calories, 9.4 grams protein, 2.2 grams carbohydrates, 5.4 grams fat, no cholesterol, and 1.4 grams dietary fiber. The same serving provides 30 percent of the RDA for magnesium (120 mg), 41 percent of the RDA for iron (6.2 mg), and 10 per-cent of the RDA for calcium (122 mg).

✤ **Selecting and storing.** Experiment with the many different varieties of soy foods. *Edamame* are soybeans in their shell, and they can be purchased in the frozen section of your grocery and stored in the pod or in the refrigerated case—cooked and out of their shells. *Tempeh* is a fermented soybean cake that has a meaty texture and can also be found in the refrigerator case. *Textured vegetable protein* (*TVP*) is processed soy that has the consistency of ground meat. It can be used in chili, sauces, soups, or anywhere you would use ground meat and is available in either the dry sec-tion of your grocery or in the freezer section. Tofu is very per-ishable and should be refrigerated for no more than a week. If it's packaged in water, drain it, cover with fresh water, and change the water daily. Tofu can be frozen for up to three months.

Culinary caution: Make sure to talk to your doctor about how much soy you should eat when trying to become pregnant and when you are pregnant.

Kitchen Prescription

All soy foods take on the flavors you cook them with, so make liberal use of those phytonutrient herbs and spices when cooking with soy products. Try our Vegetarian Chili made with textured vegetable protein for a healthy spin on a classic.

Spinach

A leafy, green native of Asia, spinach was brought to Europe by the Moors when they conquered Spain in the eighth century. Spinach contains carotenoids, folate, magnesium, iron, and calcium to support fertility and pregnancy.

✤ **Serving.** One-half cup of cooked spinach contains 21 calories, 2.7 grams protein, 3.4 grams carbohydrates, 0.2 gram fat, no cholesterol, and 2.1 grams dietary fiber. The same serving provides 74 percent of the RDA for vitamin A (737 RE), 66 percent of the RDA for folate (131.2 mcg), 20 percent of the RDA for magnesium (78.3 mg), 21 percent of the RDA for iron (3.2 mg), and 10 percent of the RDA for calcium (122.4 mg).

✤ **Selecting and storing.** Fresh spinach is available year-round. Choose leaves that are crisp and dark green with a nice fresh fragrance. Avoid those that are limp or damaged, or have yellow spots. Refrigerate in a plastic bag for up to three days.

 Kitchen Prescription

Spinach, which is usually very gritty, must be thoroughly rinsed. Get lots of it in our Spinach Lasagna.

Strawberries

The most popular American berry, more than seventy varieties of this nutrient-rich food exist. With their red color, these boisterous berries boast lycopene as one phytonutrient in their disease-fighting arsenal.

* ❖ **Serving.** One cup of raw strawberries contains 45 calories, 1 gram protein, 10.5 grams carbohydrates, 0.6 gram fat, no cholesterol, and 2.9 grams dietary fiber. The same serving provides 13 percent of the RDA for folate (26.4 mcg), 141 percent of the RDA for vitamin C (84.5 mg), 4 percent of the RDA for iron (0.6 mg), and 247 milligrams of potassium.
* ❖ **Selecting and storing.** Fresh strawberries are available year-round in many regions of the country, with the peak season from April to June. Choose brightly colored, plump berries that still have their leaves attached. Avoid soft, shriveled, or moldy berries. Do not wash until ready to use, and store in a dry container in the refrigerator for two to three days.

 Healing Tip

Stock up on frozen strawberries—or any berries, for that matter. Economical and perfect for blending into smoothies or defrosting and using as a topping for your favorite whole-grain cereal, berries are nature's perfect dessert!

Tomatoes

Thought to have originated from South America, tomatoes were brought by Spanish explorers to Europe in the 1500s. Most notable for their lycopene, tomatoes help to protect the heart by reducing oxidation of LDL cholesterol.

❖ **Serving.** One red ripe tomato (approximately 4.3 oz) contains 24 calories, 1.1 grams protein, 5.3 grams carbohydrates, 0.3 gram fat, no cholesterol, and 1.3 grams dietary fiber. The same serving provides 14 percent of the RDA for vitamin A (139 RE), 6 percent of the RDA for folate (11.6 mcg), 36 percent of the RDA for vitamin C (21.6 mg), and 5 percent of the RDA for iron (0.8 mg).

❖ **Selecting and storing.** Choose firm, well-shaped tomatoes that are fragrant and richly colored (for their variety). They should be free from blemishes, heavy for their size, and give slightly to pressure. Ripe tomatoes should be stored at room temperature and used within a few days, as cold temperatures make the flesh pithy.

 Kitchen Prescription

Cooking tomatoes helps to unlock lycopene, a fat-soluble nutrient. Adding a bit of oil also helps aid in the absorption, so get out the saucepan or try them in our Grilled Halibut with Rosemary and Tomato-Basil Sauce!

Wheat

One of the oldest grains cultivated, wheat is available in numerous forms including wheat berries, cracked wheat, bulgur grits, shredded wheat, unprocessed bran (or miller's bran), wheat germ, rolled wheat flakes, puffed wheat, cream of wheat, and wheat flour.

❖ **Serving.** One slice of whole-wheat bread contains 90 calories, 4 grams protein, 15 grams carbohydrates, 1 gram fat, no cholesterol, and 3 grams dietary fiber. The same serving provides 2 percent of the RDA for folate (4.1 mcg), 6 percent of the RDA for niacin (1.2 mg), 6 percent of the RDA for thiamin (0.09 mg), and 2 percent of the RDA for riboflavin (0.04 mg).

❖ **Selecting and storing.** Whole-wheat flour contains part of the grain's germ and turns rancid quickly because of the oil in the germ. Refrigerate or freeze these flours tightly wrapped and use as soon as possible.

 Healing Tip

Don't forget to look for the words *whole grain* when buying wheat. Whole-grain products have not been "refined" or stripped of their nutritious germ and bran layers, which help to stabilize blood sugar and fight inflammation.

So far we've looked at the nutritional elements in the spectrum of fertility-boosting foods to include in your diet every day as you work toward conception. In the next chapter, you'll learn about the nutritional requirements during pregnancy to ensure a healthy mom and baby.

Conception Accomplished: Preparing for Pregnancy

ONE-HALF OF all pregnancies are not planned! This means it's important for a woman to have her body in pregnancy-bearing health as she works to accomplish conception. After reading the earlier chapters, you're hopefully eating to enhance fertility with blood-sugar-balancing carbs and fats, healthy sources of protein, and a bevy of pregnancy-boosting antioxidant phytonutrients. However, at this stage, it's also important for a woman to ensure that she is conscious of the nutrients needed to support pregnancy, and prevent birth defects and complications. In this chapter, we'll discuss prenatal nutrition as well as the body changes, cravings, and culinary cautions to keep in mind during pregnancy.

Prenatal Nutrition: Vitamins and Minerals

As a woman gears up toward pregnancy, it's important that she has her body prepared for the next nine months. While her diet should provide her with the nutrition needed to support herself and her growing baby during pregnancy, women trying to become pregnant are advised to take prenatal vitamins. Specially formulated, these multivitamins make up for any nutritional deficiencies in the diet during pregnancy. A woman should talk with her doctor about a prenatal vitamin that's right, containing approximately:

* ❖ 4,000 to 5,000 RE of vitamin A
* ❖ 800 to 1,000 micrograms (1 mg) of folate
* ❖ 400 IU of vitamin D
* ❖ 200 to 300 milligrams of calcium
* ❖ 75 milligrams of vitamin C
* ❖ 1.5 milligrams of thiamin
* ❖ 1.6 milligrams of riboflavin
* ❖ 2.6 milligrams of pyridoxine
* ❖ 17 milligrams of niacinamide
* ❖ 2.2 milligrams of vitamin B_{12}
* ❖ 10 milligrams of vitamin E
* ❖ 15 milligrams of zinc
* ❖ 30 milligrams of iron

In addition, the following nutrients and foods will help to ensure optimum health for Mom and Baby.

Folate

Neural tube defects develop in the first twenty-eight days after conception, and folic acid (or folate) can help prevent these problems. If a woman doesn't get enough folic acid, the baby's spine may not form right—a condition called *spina bifida*—or his brain may not form or only partly form—a condition called *anencephaly* (an-en-seffelee).

Before a woman gets pregnant and in the first three months while she's pregnant, she should try to get 400 micrograms (or 0.4 mg) of folate daily from foods fortified with folate or a vitamin or folate pill. Many doctors recommend a vitamin that has folate, but vitamins or folate pills are available at the drugstore or grocery store. A woman could get her folate though food alone, but it is hard to know if she's getting enough, so taking it in a pill is the best way to be sure she's getting the right amount. However, a healthy diet is always good for Mom and Baby.

Healing Tip

Get folate in black-eyed peas (105 mcg or 25 percent DV), cooked spinach (100 mcg or 25 percent DV), great northern beans (90 mcg or 20 percent DV), asparagus (85 mcg or 20 percent DV), wheat germ (40 mcg or 10 percent DV), orange juice (35 mcg or 10 percent DV), peas (50 mcg or 15 percent DV), cooked broccoli (45 mcg or 15 percent), avocados (45 mcg or 10 percent DV), and peanuts (40 mcg or 10 percent DV).

Calcium

A baby needs calcium for strong bones and teeth, so plenty of calcium-rich foods—such as nonfat or low-fat yogurt and milk and broccoli should be eaten. Your physician may recommend additional calcium supplements when pregnant and breast-feeding.

Healing Tip

Get calcium in low-fat yogurt (415 mg or 42 percent DV), sardines (245 mg or 25 percent DV), cheddar cheese (306 mg or 31 percent DV), nonfat milk (402 mg or 30 percent DV), tofu (204 mg or 20 percent DV), fortified orange juice (200 mg or 20 percent DV), canned salmon with bones (181 mg or 18 percent DV), cottage cheese (138 mg or 14 percent DV), and cooked spinach (120 mg or 12 percent DV).

Iron

The mom-to-be needs iron to keep her blood healthy for herself and her baby. Bones and teeth also need iron to develop properly, and too little iron can cause a condition called *anemia*. If Mom has anemia, she might look pale and feel very tired. Her doctor can check for signs of anemia through the routine blood tests that are taken in different stages of the pregnancy.

All pregnant women should take a low-dose iron supplement, beginning at the first prenatal visit (or even before when she is planning to get pregnant). Prenatal vitamins that a doctor prescribes or that are found over-the-counter usually have the amount of iron needed; however, check the label to make sure they contain iron. If the doctor finds that she has anemia, he or she will give a higher dose of iron supplements to take once or twice a day.

There are two forms of dietary iron: *heme* and *nonheme*. Heme iron is derived from hemoglobin, the protein in red blood cells that delivers oxygen to cells. Heme iron is found in animal foods that originally contained hemoglobin, such as red meats, fish, and poultry. Iron in plant foods such as lentils and beans is arranged in a chemical structure called *nonheme iron*. This is the form of iron added to iron-enriched and iron-fortified foods. Although heme iron is absorbed better than nonheme iron, by eating veggie-based sources of iron with some vitamin C, it will boost absorption.

Healing Tip

Get iron in ready-to-eat iron fortified cereal (18 mg or 100 percent DV), fortified oatmeal (10 mg or 60 percent DV), soybeans (8 mg or 50 percent DV), lentils (6.6 mg or 35 percent DV), kidney beans (5.2 mg or 25 percent DV), lima beans (4.5 mg or 25 percent DV), navy beans (4.5 mg or 20 percent DV), black beans (3.6 mg or 20 percent DV), pinto beans (3.6 mg or 20 percent DV), tofu (3.4 mg or 20 percent DV), cooked spinach (3.2 mg or 20 percent DV), white meat turkey (1.6 mg or 8 percent DV), and chicken breast (1.1 mg or 6 percent DV).

Fat

Avoid eating a lot of foods high in saturated fat (such as butter and fatty meats). Instead, choose leaner foods when you can (such as skim milk, chicken and turkey without the skin, and fish). In addition, opt for the healthy fats we talked about in Chapter 3, which include the PUFAs and MUFAs. Omega-3 fats are especially important in your baby's health development.

 Healing Tip

Get healthy fats in raw, unsalted nuts and seeds, low-mercury fish (see Chapter 3 under omega-3 fats and also in "Culinary Cautions" at the end of this chapter), avocados, and vegetable oils including extra-virgin olive oil.

Fruits, Veggies, and Legumes

Eat seven or more servings of fruits and vegetables (a minimum of three servings of fruit and four of vegetables) daily for vitamins, minerals, phytonutrients, and fiber.

Healing Tip

✢ One serving size of fruit equals 1 medium apple, 1 medium banana, ½ cup of chopped fruit, or ¾ cup of fruit juice.
✢ One serving size vegetable equals 1 cup raw leafy vegetables, ½ cup of other vegetables (raw or cooked), or ¾ cup vegetable juice.

Whole Grains

Whole-grain products and enriched products such as bread, rice, pasta, and breakfast cereals contain iron, B vitamins, some protein, minerals, and fiber that your body needs. In addition, some breakfast cereals have been enriched with 100 percent of the folate your body needs each day, which as we discussed previously, has been shown to help prevent some serious birth defects. Choosing a breakfast cereal or other enriched grain products that contain folate is important before and during pregnancy.

Healing Tip

One serving size of grains equals 1 slice bread; ½ cup of cooked cereal, rice, or pasta; or 1 cup ready-to-eat cereal.

Dairy

As we mentioned earlier, Mom and Baby need calcium for strong bones and teeth. Dairy products also have vitamins A and D, protein, and B vitamins. Vitamin A helps growth, resistance to infection, and vision. Aim for four or more servings of low-fat or nonfat milk, yogurt, or other dairy products such as cheese for calcium, as pregnant women need 1,000 milligrams of calcium each day. For women eighteen or younger, aim for 1,300 milligrams of calcium each day. Choosing low-fat or non-fat milk and milk products helps to lower fat intake. Other sources of calcium include dark green leafy vegetables, dried beans and peas, nuts and seeds, and tofu.

If the mom-to-be is lactose intolerant or can't digest dairy products, she can still get this extra calcium. There are several low-lactose or reduced-lactose products available as well as calcium-fortified soy milk, if her doctor recommends it. In some cases, a doctor might advise her to take a calcium supplement.

 Healing Tip

Go Organic! Organic dairy products are produced without the use of hormones or antibiotics. One serving size of dairy equals 1 cup of milk or yogurt or 1½ ounces natural cheese. Don't forget, women who are pregnant should not consume soft, unpasteurized cheeses including feta, goat, Brie, Camembert, and blue cheese (discussed in "Culinary Cautions" at the end of the chapter).

Protein

Protein builds muscle, tissue, enzymes, hormones, and antibodies for Mom and Baby. These foods also have B vitamins and iron, which is important for red blood cells. Pregnant women need about 60 grams of protein per day. This is about the same as two or more 2- to 3-ounce servings of cooked lean meat, poultry without the skin or fish, or two or more 1-ounce servings of cooked meat. Eggs, nuts, dried beans, and peas also are good forms of protein, and most women in this country have no problem getting at least this amount of protein each day.

The need for protein in the first trimester is small but grows in the second and third trimesters when the baby is growing the fastest and Mom's body is working to meet her growing needs.

 Healing Tip

One serving size of protein equals 2 to 3 ounces of cooked lean meat, poultry, or fish; ½ cup cooked dried beans; 1 egg; ½ cup tofu; ⅓ cup nuts; or 2 tablespoons peanut butter. Remember, don't eat uncooked or undercooked meats, fish, or eggs; and avoid deli luncheon meats, hot dogs, and cold cuts. (See "Culinary Cautions" at the end of the chapter for more info.)

Water

Water plays a key role in your diet during pregnancy. It carries the nutrients from the foods to the baby and helps prevent constipation, hemorrhoids, excessive swelling, and urinary tract or bladder infections. Drinking enough water, especially in the last trimester, also helps prevent dehydration. Not getting enough water can then lead to having contractions and premature or early labor.

Pregnant women should drink at least eight 8-ounce glasses of water per day and another glass for each hour of activity. Mom can drink juices for fluid, but they also have a lot of calories and can cause extra weight gain.

Healing Tip

Coffee, soft drinks, and teas that have caffeine actually reduce the amount of fluid in your body, so they cannot count toward the total amount of fluid you need.

During Pregnancy

The following tips will help Mom achieve a lifestyle that will gear her body toward optimum health in these critical nine months.

✤ **Tell your doctor if you smoke or use alcohol or drugs.** Quitting is hard, but you can do it. Ask your doctor for help.

✤ **Get enough sleep.** Try to get seven to nine hours every night.

✤ **If you can, control the stress in your life.** When it comes to things like work and family, figure out what you can really do. Set limits with yourself and others. Don't be afraid to say no to requests for your time and energy.

✤ **Move your body.** Once you get pregnant, it's difficult to increase your exercise routine by a lot, so it's best to start before the baby is on the way.

✤ **Get any health problems under control.** Talk to your doctor about how your health problems might affect you and your baby while pregnant. If you have diabetes, monitor your blood sugar levels. If you have high blood pressure, monitor these levels as well. If you are overweight, talk to your doctor about what a healthy weight is for you. In addition, get checked for hepatitis B and C, sexually transmitted diseases (STDs), and HIV, and tell your doctor if you or your sex partners have ever had an STD or HIV, since these can harm both you and your baby.

❖ **Find out what health problems run in your family.** Tell these to your doctor so you can get genetic testing for some health problems that might run in your family. In addition, ask your mother, aunts, grandmothers, and sisters about their pregnancies. Did they have morning sickness? Problems with labor? How did they cope with them?

❖ **Make sure you have had all of your immunizations (shots).** One immunization that is especially important is rubella (German measles). If you haven't had chickenpox or rubella, get the shots at least three months before getting pregnant.

❖ **Go over all of the medicines you take (prescriptions, OTCs, and herbals) with your doctor.** Ask her if they are safe to take while you are trying to get pregnant or are pregnant.

Eating Twice as Smart, Not Twice as Much

While pregnant, a woman will need additional nutrients to keep her and her baby healthy. However, that doesn't mean she needs to eat twice as much. She should increase her caloric intake by about 300 calories per day, but she should make sure not to restrict her diet during pregnancy, which can prohibit her from getting the right amounts of protein, vitamins, and minerals that are necessary to properly nourish the baby. Low-calorie intake can cause a pregnant mother's stored fat to break down, leading to the production of substances called *ketones*. Ketones, which can be found in the mother's blood and urine, are a sign of starvation or a starvation-like state. Constant production of ketones can severely impact the development of your child.

Managing Morning Sickness

Morning sickness and nausea are common problems for pregnant women. Most nausea occurs during the early part of pregnancy and, in most cases, will subside once she enters the second trimester. For some women, morning sickness and nausea might last longer than the early stages of pregnancy or even throughout the entire nine months.

The changes in her body might cause her to be nauseated or to vomit when she smells or eats certain things, when she is tired or stressed, or for no apparent reason at all. Nausea in early pregnancy is a condition that often can be managed by changing when and what she eats. Here are some tips for the mom-to-be struggling with nausea:

❖ Eat smaller meals each day, such as six to eight small meals instead of three larger ones.
❖ Avoid being without food for long periods of time.
❖ Drink fluids between, but not with, meals.
❖ Avoid foods that are greasy, fried, or highly spiced.
❖ Avoid foul and unpleasant odors.
❖ Rest when you are tired.

Severe nausea and vomiting in pregnancy are rare, but if they occur, they can cause dehydration, which can require medical attention. In severe cases, Mom should immediately go to the hospital or see her physician. If she feels that nausea or vomiting is keeping her from eating right or gaining enough weight, she should talk with her doctor and ask about the safety of drinking ginger tea or eating ginger candy.

Dealing with Body Changes and Weight Gain

During a pregnancy, weight should be gained gradually, with most of the weight gained in the last trimester. Good rates of weight gain are about two to four pounds during the first three months of pregnancy and three to four pounds per month for the rest of the pregnancy. The average total weight gain should be about twenty-five to thirty pounds, but the amount gained might be slightly less or more—depending on Mom's height and weight before she became pregnant. According to the American College of Obstetricians and Gynecologists (ACOG), if a woman was underweight before becoming pregnant, she should gain between twenty-eight and forty pounds; if she was overweight before becoming pregnant, she should gain between fifteen and twenty-five pounds. It's best for the mom-to-be to check with her doctor to find out how much weight gain during pregnancy is healthy for her.

Although it varies from woman to woman, let's take a look at where the weight comes from:

* 7.5 pounds—average baby's weight
* 7 pounds—your body's extra stored protein, fat, and other nutrients
* 4 pounds—your extra blood
* 4 pounds—your other extra body fluids
* 2 pounds—breast enlargement
* 2 pounds—enlargement of your uterus
* 2 pounds—amniotic fluid surrounding your baby
* 1.5 pounds—the placenta

Total weight gained during pregnancy includes six to eight pounds for the weight of the baby. The remaining weight consists of a higher fluid volume, larger breasts, larger uterus, amniotic fluid, and the placenta. Make sure to visit your doctor throughout your pregnancy so she can check on your weight gain.

It can be hard to lose weight after you have your baby if you gained too much weight during pregnancy. During pregnancy, fat deposits can increase by more than one-third of the total amount you had before becoming pregnant. If weight gain during pregnancy is normal, most women lose this extra weight in the birth process and in the weeks and months after birth. Recent research shows that women who gain more than the recommended amount during pregnancy and who fail to lose this weight within six months after giving birth are at much higher risk of being obese nearly ten years later. Breast-feeding also can help to deplete the fat gained during pregnancy by helping the body to expend at least 500 more calories each day. For more information on diet and nutrition while breast-feeding go to the website 4woman.gov/breastfeeding/print-bf.cfm?page=235.

Handling Cravings

Changes in nutritional needs may be the culprit of the "pickles and ice cream" choices and other appetite cravings of pregnant women. The fetus needs nourishment, and the mother's body begins to absorb and metabolize nutrients differently. These changes help ensure normal development of the baby and fill the demands of lactation, or breast-feeding, after the baby is born.

Some pregnant women crave chocolate, spicy foods, fruits, and comfort foods—such as mashed potatoes and cereals. Other women crave non-food items—such as clay and cornstarch. The craving and eating of non-food items are known as *pica*, and consuming things that aren't food can be dangerous to both Mom and Baby. If a woman has urges to eat non-food items, she should notify her doctor.

Culinary Cautions

Making sure Mom eats the right foods and amounts during pregnancy is only one part of proper nutrition. It is also important that she watches out for and avoids these culinary cautions to ensure a safe and healthy pregnancy.

Alcohol and Caffeine During Pregnancy

There is no safe time during pregnancy for you to drink alcohol, and there is no known safe amount of alcohol to drink during pregnancy. When a pregnant woman drinks beer, wine, hard liquor, or other alcoholic beverages, alcohol gets into her blood and is transferred to her baby through the umbilical cord. When the alcohol enters his body, it can slow down his growth, affect his brain, and cause birth defects. *Fetal alcohol spectrum disorders* (*FASD*) is a broad term describing the range of effects that can occur in a person whose mother drank alcohol during pregnancy. Some people with FASD may have abnormal facial features and growth and central nervous system problems. People with FASD may also have problems with learning, memory, attention span, communication, vision, and/or hearing; these problems often lead to issues in school and with behavior. The effects of FASD last a lifetime. Moms-to-be: if you are pregnant and have been drinking alcohol, stop drinking now to protect your baby. If you need help to stop drinking, talk with your doctor or nurse. For more information go to the website 4woman .gov/faq/fas.htm.

Caffeine is a stimulant found in colas, coffee, tea, chocolate, cocoa, and some over-the-counter and prescription drugs. Consumed in large quantities, caffeine can cause irritability, nervousness, and insomnia as well as low-birth-weight babies. Caffeine is also a diuretic and can dehydrate a woman's body of valuable water. Some studies show that caffeine intake during pregnancy can harm the fetus; so until more is known, you should avoid caffeine. In addition, caffeine is an ingredient in many over-the-counter and prescription drugs, so Moms, talk with your doctor before taking any drugs or medicines while pregnant.

Fish, Meat, Dairy, and Other Protein Foods to Avoid During Pregnancy

As we discussed in Chapter 3, it is advisable for pregnant women to stay away from the following specific varieties of fish during pregnancy because of methylmercury:

❖ Shark
❖ Swordfish
❖ King mackerel
❖ Tuna (albacore)

However, moms-to-be may eat up to 12 ounces (two average meals) a week of a variety of fish and shellfish that are lower in mercury. Five of the most commonly eaten fish that are low in mercury are shrimp, canned light tuna, salmon, pollack, and catfish. Albacore (white) tuna has more mercury than canned light tuna. When choosing meals of fish and shellfish, pregnant women may eat up to six ounces, one average meal, of albacore tuna per week.

Because of the estrogenic effects of soy, a pregnant woman should talk with her doctor about how much soy is safe to incorporate during pregnancy and the specific types to include.

In addition, being aware of specific bacteria present in and around foods and their risk factors is especially important in pregnancy. Salmonella species, *Helicobacter pylori*, shigella, *Escherichia coli* (E. coli), cryptosporidium, *Listeria monocytogenes*, and *Toxoplasma gondii* are some of the culprits of food-borne illness that affect pregnant women. Processed meats are high in saturated fat and contain preservatives that are unhealthy for Mom and Baby. In general, it is important for moms-to-be to stay away from:

- Unpasteurized milk products (including feta, Brie, and Camembert and blue-veined and Mexican-style cheeses)
- Unpasteurized juices
- Raw meats, fish, shellfish, and poultry products
- Processed meats, deli meat, cold cuts, hot dogs
- Raw sprouts
- Unwashed fruits and veggies (always wash well!)

Now that you are armed with the foods and nutrients for boosting fertility and having a healthy pregnancy, in this next chapter, we offer shopping tips for getting these important foods into your pantry so you can *eat your medicine*!

8

The Pregnancy Pantry: Shopping for Health

IN YOUR GOAL to balance blood sugar, reduce inflammation, boost fertility, and have a healthy pregnancy, your first step is to choose the right ingredients. Unfortunately, with so many products on the market, selecting healthful items to stock your pantry can be a daunting task. In this chapter, we give you practical tips on deciphering food labels and the art of shopping for health.

Strategies for Smart Shopping

Understanding the science behind how foods can protect us is only useful if we can translate that information into our grocery carts and ultimately onto our tables. Because most of us spend a substantial amount of time at the grocery (84 percent of consumers prepare home-cooked meals at least three times a week), it is critical to navigate the supermarket smorgasbord to sleuth out the healthiest products.

Before you go to the store, make a list, check it twice. Smart shopping begins before you leave the house. Being unprepared leads to multiple trips and unwanted, often unhealthy, items finding their way into your shopping cart. Instead of buying on impulse, stray from your list only if the item is a healthy one. If a junior shopper vying for the candy aisle accompanies you, have him or her explore the produce section and choose a unique fruit or vegetable to try (e.g., a persimmon, pomegranate, or a kiwi). Also, before you venture to the grocery store, you should eat first. Shopping hungry is a surefire way to end up straying from your list and succumbing to unhealthy choices. Having a small snack will help you to avoid temptations that will wind up in your cupboard and on your waist.

When filling your cart, become a perimeter shopper. The exterior of the store contains many of the whole foods we have described for optimum health. Spend most of your time shopping for fresh produce, seafood, lean meats, and dairy. When choosing dairy, opt for lower calorie products, such as shredded mozzarella; fresh, soft cheeses; and yogurt as opposed to aged, hard cheeses like cheddar—which rack up 100 calories for each one-ounce cube. And remember, pregnant women should choose pasteurized cheese.

There is so much variation in the health value of different brands of foods, so it's important to pause, read labels, and compare choices. Read ingredient lists, and look at calories and sugar, the type of grain used (whole grains versus refined), and the type of oils used (partially hydrogenated palm kernel oil versus olive oil). We will demystify the food label later in this chapter.

Filling Your Cart

It's easy to incorporate all the fertility-boosting foods, plus the good fats and good carbs we talked about in earlier chapters. Remember those colors we described in Chapter 6? You want to look for those same colors to put them in your cart and build your meals around them. When you look in your shopping cart, the vast majority of your food selection should be fruits and vegetables to reach the goal of at least five to nine servings a day. Blue blueberry smoothies, hearty red marinara sauces, green salads, and multicolored vegetable soups should be your mainstays.

Frozen vegetables, fruits, seafood, and poultry are an economical and convenient way to eat healthy. Having a freezer stocked with these staples ensures you can whip up a delicious meal in minutes. Here are some ideas to get you started.

* Try frozen fruits like blueberries, mixed berries, or cherries for the smoothies and fruit-based desserts that we provide in Chapter 10.
* Opt for frozen edamame (soybeans in their pods) for an easy appetizer for an Asian meal.
* Bagged, mixed veggies are perfect to make vegetable soups, and research shows that the nutrient content is equal to or greater than fresh foods, which can lose many vitamins in the shipping and handling.

By adding a few additional ingredients, frozen foods can provide you with a healthy base for many of your meals.

Buy high-quality cooking oils such as extra-virgin olive oil, sesame oil, canola oil, and other liquid vegetable oils for sautéing or making dressings and marinades. Buy mustard, vinegars, horseradish, and the dried herbs and spices that add virtually no calories and lots of flavor and unique phytonutrients to all varieties of foods.

Finally, go nuts for your health! Instead of chips, pretzels, and other nutrient-void snack foods, opt for raw nuts and seeds, which are full of minerals, good-quality fats, and many other health-promoting nutrients. Just be sure to watch your portion size, as a quarter cup of almonds contains 170 calories.

Buyer Beware: What to Watch Out For

Beware of not-so-healthy "health" foods. Sports drinks and energy bars are not much more than sugar fortified with vitamins and minerals, each packing a whopping 200-plus calories per serving. The same goes for desserts and snack foods that are labeled "organic." These are no better than their conventional counterparts when it comes to nutrition.

Remember how we talked about the dangers of processed meats and red meats and their negative effects on fertility, dangers to the developing fetus in pregnancy, and general health in Chapters 3 and 7? It's a good idea to avoid the deli when shopping. Although many deli foods are marketed as "fresh," most are processed red meats or poultry.

Finally, don't drown in the beverage aisle. Other than good old H_2O, there's nothing in the beverage aisle you want to buy. This also goes for sugary, high-calorie iced teas; pseudo-smoothies; sweetened milks; and coffee beverages. Don't be deterred by teas, though, which provide a spectrum of antioxidant phytonutrients and help to balance blood sugar.

Understanding Label Lingo

Just about every packaged food made in the United States has a food label indicating serving size, nutritional information, and ingredients. Unfortunately, this critical piece of information is often overlooked, leading to unhealthy food choices that could have easily been avoided. The very first thing you should do when deciding on a product is look at the ingredient list. This is the most detailed information on what a product contains and can help to answer the following questions.

❖ **Are the fats used in this product healthful or harmful?** Remember to look for foods made with olive, canola, or other healthful oils and avoid partially hydrogenated oils. This is of particular concern for packaged cereals, cookies, crackers, microwave popcorn, pastry, cake mixes, chips, and other cereal products; it also applies to soups, frozen foods, and other premade convenience foods. (Refer back to Chapter 3 to learn about your friends and foes of the fat world.)

❖ **Is the product made with whole grains?** As we mentioned previously, good carbs help to balance blood sugar. If the label does not say "whole," the product is made with refined flour. Instead of "wheat" flour, for example, look for "whole-wheat" flour. This also applies for all other grains.

❖ **How much of each ingredient does the product contain?** The ingredient list is in descending order. The farther down the list you go, the less of that ingredient the product contains.

❖ **Is the product full of sugar?** Avoid products with high fructose corn syrup, as well as fruit sweeteners appearing high on the ingredient list. Although sugars from fruits in nature may be more healthful when consumed in their natural state (e.g., as part of that Red Delicious apple), juice concentrate sweeteners have the same effect on blood sugar and same number of calories as pure sugar.

❖ **How much of the product is a fruit or vegetable?** Although the product may be called "Strawberry Crunchies," after reading the food label you may find only a trace of strawberry flavor toward the end of the list. Choose foods that are nutrient dense and stay away from those that are merely empty calories.

Examining Serving Size

Serving sizes are based on the amount of food people typically eat. However, many products contain multiple servings per package. Individual snack foods, for example, may contain 100 calories per serving, but when you read the number of servings, you find that energy bar you just ate contains three servings at 100 calories per serving, totaling 300 calories, as opposed to the 100 you may have assumed. It not only affects calories but also the amounts of all other nutritional components like fat, sugar, and salt.

Examining Calories and Total Fat

Look at calories and focus on where they come from. Use your calories as you would a daily stipend and try to make the most of each. Are your calories coming from good-quality fats and whole grains, or are they derived from sugars or saturated and trans fats?

The total fat panel provides the total amount of fat per serving and also breaks down the amount and type of each. You can decipher how much trans fat is in a product with a simple math equation.

By adding the saturated fat, monounsaturated fat, and polyunsaturated fats and subtracting them from the total fat, you will determine the grams of trans fat in a specific product. For example, look at Smart Balance Popcorn. The total fat is 9 grams. The saturated fat is 3.5 grams, the monounsaturated fat is 2.5 grams, and the polyunsaturated fat is 3 grams.

9 − (3.5 grams saturated fat + 2.5 grams monounsaturated fat + 3 grams polyunsaturated fat) = 0 grams trans fat

Talk with your doctor regarding what percentage of calories in your diet should come from fat, depending on your particular nutrition needs.

Examining Cholesterol Content

Dietary cholesterol can raise your blood cholesterol level, although usually not as much as saturated fat or trans fat. Because dietary cholesterol is found only in foods that come from animals, by choosing plenty of fruits, vegetables, and whole grains, you can stay under the daily 300 milligrams recommended by the American Heart Association.

A Look at Label Claims

Another aspect of food labeling is label claims. Three types of claims can be used for foods and dietary supplements: health claims, nutrient content claims, and structure/function claims.

Health claims describe a relationship between a food, food component, or dietary supplement ingredient and its effect on reducing the risk of a particular disease or health-related condition.

Nutrient content claims characterize the level of nutrient in a food product using terms such as *free, light,* and *low,* or they compare the level of a nutrient in a food to that of another food, using terms such as *more, reduced,* or *light.* These requirements ensure that terms are used consistently for all products and are useful to consumers. However, it's important to appreciate that sometimes the so-called "good" and "excellent" sources of nutrients may not be consistent or uniformly defined. This will give you a practical tool to help make sound nutritional choices regarding diet.

Structure and *function claims* describe the role of a nutrient or dietary ingredient intended to affect normal structure or function in humans. Examples of structure/function claims include "calcium builds strong bones," "fiber maintains bowel regularity," and "antioxidants maintain cell integrity." You will find these types of claims on functional foods that may be fortified, such as fiber laxatives and some supplements.

Now that you're armed with powerful information on the healing nutrients of certain foods it's time to put all of this information to use in the delicious and healthy meal plans and recipes courtesy of Healing Gourmet. Bon appétit!

9

My Daily Dose: Meal Plans to Get You Started

YOU DON'T HAVE to be a master chef to be a Healing Gourmet. Just let the principles and recipes in this book guide you. We have included recipes suited for the culinary novice, those pressed for time, and those who want to maintain their healthy weight or lose weight—and we do it without sacrificing any flavor. Mealtime should be one of the most enjoyable of your day, so let us help you to make it healthy!

In this section you will find seven-day meal plans for three different calorie levels—1,600, 2,000, and 2,400 calories. We recognize that readers will have different goals for their overall nutrition. These meal plans are only intended for use as a guide or template for meals and snacks. The right calorie level for an individual depends on his or her height, age, activity level, and goals for nutrition. For example, if you are carrying excess weight or are currently inactive, you may consider the 1,600-calorie menu. On the other hand, if you are active and have a healthy body weight, the 2,000- or 2,400-calorie menus may work for you. To help select an appropriate calorie level for you, we recommend you schedule an appointment with your registered dietitian or physician.

Each of these meal plans incorporates the science of good nutrition that you've just read about into practical, flavorful, and easy-to-prepare recipes you can put together for yourself or your family. However, no matter what your calorie level is, each of these calorie levels incorporates the following healthy principles of diet planning:

❖ Use a variety of *lean protein sources* (averaging 20 to 25 percent of calories)—limiting high fatty cuts of meat, incorporating fish, and encouraging meatless meals throughout the week.
❖ Emphasize *healthy fats* (using monounsaturated and polyunsaturated fats as a primary fat source—averaging 22 to 30 percent of total calories).
❖ Incorporate *healthy, whole-grain carbohydrates* (averaging 50 to 60 percent of total calories) for optimal blood sugar control.

They all limit or avoid the following:

❖ Saturated fats—averaging less than 7 percent of calories
❖ Trans fats
❖ Dietary cholesterol—most days no more than 300 milligrams per day (If you have high cholesterol, aim for 200 or less)
❖ Sodium—most days less than 2,400 milligrams

Finally, all these meal plans encourage:

❖ A variety of foods—especially fruits, vegetables, and whole grains (Remember: go for a variety of color and texture in your food choices.)

✤ Eating plenty of fruits and vegetables

✤ Using whole grains as the main choice for breads, cereals, crackers, and pasta

✤ High fiber—with a minimum of 25 grams per day

✤ Using whole foods, free-range poultry, locally grown produce, and fresh herbs and spices

Throughout the chapter, you'll find meals for breakfast, lunch, and dinner, as well as snacks to eat throughout the day. We also include information about the nutritional content for the day and feature recipes from Chapter 10 (indicated with an asterisk*). Our *Veg Out* option features a vegetarian alternative for dinner; non-meat eaters can also find more vegetarian lunch options for the meat-filled lunches in our soup and salad section in the recipe chapter. Please note if you select the *Veg Out* option, the calories and other nutrients (protein, fat, carbohydrate, etc.) will vary somewhat from the meal plan. In addition, we recommend drinking six to eight glasses of water a day. You can substitute low-sodium sparkling water for two of the six glasses a day and spring water with a lemon wedge to add some variety.

My Meal Plans: 1,600 Calories

If you are trying to have a baby or are pregnant but hold excess body weight, this calorie plan may be just the one for you. It ensures you get optimal fertility-boosting nutrients and phytonutrients without excess calories. Your doctor can tell you if this plan may be right for you.

Day 1

Breakfast
½ cup old-fashioned oats (prepared with water)
½ cup frozen unsweetened blueberries
¼ cup nonfat plain yogurt topped with
2 tablespoons ground walnuts

Midmorning Snack
1 cup decaffeinated black tea with ½ teaspoon cinnamon
6 ounces nonfat light yogurt

Lunch
3 ounces canned chicken in water, drained
3 cups fresh baby spinach
¼ cup sliced red onion
¼ cup sliced mushrooms
4 cherry tomatoes
2 tablespoons light vinaigrette salad dressing
1 sprouted grain roll

Midafternoon Snack
1 medium apple
1½ ounces part-skim mozzarella cheese
Cinnamon apple tea

Dinner
1 serving Vegetarian Chili* topped with
¼ cup 2 percent fat shredded cheddar cheese and
2 tablespoons light sour cream
1 cup steamed broccoli, cauliflower, and carrots
1 ounce whole-grain crackers

SNACK
½ cup low-fat vanilla frozen yogurt
½ cup sliced strawberries
Herbal tea

What's inside? 1,560 calories, 89 grams protein, 194 grams carbohydrates, 56 grams total fat, 17 grams saturated fat, 85 milligrams cholesterol, 2,370 milligrams sodium, 35 grams dietary fiber

---

Day 2

BREAKFAST
Two Kashi Go Lean frozen waffles topped with
½ medium banana
1 1.3-ounce vegetarian sausage patty
Decaffeinated coffee

MIDMORNING SNACK
1 cup herbal tea or cinnamon apple tea
1 medium orange

LUNCH
Homemade "pizza": in toaster oven heat one small whole-wheat
   pita topped with 2 ounces marinara sauce, 2 ounces part-skim
   mozzarella cheese, and 1 cup sliced red, yellow, and green
   peppers
2 tablespoons light ranch dressing to dip

MIDAFTERNOON SNACK
6 ounces nonfat light fruit yogurt
Low-sodium mineral water

DINNER
1 serving Mussels Fra Diavolo*
1 cup steamed broccoli topped with
1 tablespoon grated Parmesan cheese

Veg Out! *Try our Spinach Lasagna for a meatless meal with Italian appeal.*

SNACK
¼ cup unsalted soy nuts
2 tablespoons dried unsweetened cranberries
Cinnamon apple tea

What's inside? 1,580 calories, 108 grams protein, 186 grams carbohydrates, 45 grams total fat, 12 grams saturated fat, 145 milligrams cholesterol, 3,160 milligrams sodium, 30 grams dietary fiber

Day 3

BREAKFAST
1 cup shredded wheat cereal topped with
1 cup skim milk and
2 tablespoons raisins
Decaffeinated coffee

MIDMORNING SNACK
Wedges of one grapefruit
6 ounces light nonfat yogurt
Orange spice tea

LUNCH
2 servings Pea in the Pod Soup*
1 small whole-wheat pita
½ cup 1 percent fat cottage cheese

MIDAFTERNOON SNACK
½ ounce dry-roasted almonds
Low-sodium sparkling water

DINNER
4 ounces baked tilapia
2 cups steamed green beans
1 small sweet potato
2 teaspoons trans fat–free tub margarine

Veg Out! *Try our Summer Ratatouille for a refreshing vegetarian twist.*

SNACK
5 ginger snap cookies
8 ounces chocolate soy milk

What's inside? 1,560 calories, 95 grams protein, 234 grams carbohydrates, 34 grams total fat, 5 grams saturated fat, 100 milligrams cholesterol, 1,850 milligrams sodium, 35 grams dietary fiber

---

Day 4

BREAKFAST
1 whole-wheat English muffin, toasted under broiler or in
   toaster oven, topped with
½ cup 1 percent fat cottage cheese and
¾ cup sliced strawberries and ¼ teaspoon cinnamon
1 cup decaffeinated coffee with nonfat creamer

MIDMORNING SNACK
2 whole-wheat graham crackers topped with
2 teaspoons almond butter

LUNCH
1 large ripe tomato cored and stuffed with
¼ cup brown rice,
2 ounces diced chicken,
2 tablespoons light mayonnaise, and
Diced celery and onion
5 reduced-fat, woven-wheat crackers
1 medium apple

MIDAFTERNOON SNACK
1 string cheese
Decaffeinated green tea with lemon

DINNER
1 serving Penne with Spring Vegetables*
1 cup tossed salad topped with
1 tablespoon light vinaigrette dressing

SNACK
Orange spice tea

What's inside? 1,590 calories, 80 grams protein, 216 grams
carbohydrates, 52 grams total fat, 11 grams saturated fat, 85 grams
cholesterol, 2,680 milligrams sodium, 30 grams dietary fiber

Day 5

BREAKFAST
1 serving Mixed Berry Scones*
1 serving Chocolate and Peanut Butter Smoothie*

MIDMORNING SNACK
1 medium pear
½ cup 1 percent fat cottage cheese

LUNCH
3 cups tossed salad greens combined with
¼ cup shredded carrots,
¼ cup sliced cucumbers,
¼ cup diced celery,
2 ounces baked barbecue flavored tofu, and
2 tablespoons light salad dressing
1 ounce whole-wheat pretzels

MIDAFTERNOON SNACK
1 cup cut-up fresh vegetables
¼ cup red pepper hummus
Herbal tea

DINNER
4 ounces roast turkey
One small baked potato with skin topped with
¼ cup fresh salsa
2 cups steamed spinach and red peppers

Veg Out! *Enjoy our Veggie Burgers with a side of Cabbage and Apple Slaw for a picnic-perfect meal!*

SNACK
1 cup diced fresh melon
Decaffeinated black tea with ½ teaspoon cinnamon

What's inside? 1,560 calories, 99 grams protein, 188 grams carbohydrates, 44 grams total fat, 6 grams saturated fat, 100 milligrams cholesterol, 2,860 milligrams sodium, 38 grams dietary fiber

Day 6

BREAKFAST
½ cup Swiss Muesli* topped with
6 ounces (¾ cup) skim milk and
¼ cup fresh raspberries
Green tea

MIDMORNING SNACK
½ ounce unsalted dry-roasted peanuts
Herbal tea

LUNCH
1 cup Spinach Leek Soup*
1 slice cracked-wheat bread topped with
3 ounces lemon pepper turkey breast, lettuce, tomato, and
2 teaspoons Dijon mustard
1 medium apple

MIDAFTERNOON SNACK
3 cups low-fat, reduced-sodium microwave popcorn
8 ounces sparkling water with wedge of lime

DINNER
1 serving Chicken with Quinoa and Garbanzo Beans*
1½ cups tossed mixed greens topped with
¼ cup sliced radish
¼ cup sliced carrot
¼ cup diced celery
2 tablespoons balsamic vinaigrette dressing
Spring water

Veg Out! *Complement our Rice, Bean, and Mango Salad with your favorite Veggie Burger for a meal in minutes!*

Snack
1 cup no-sugar-added hot chocolate

What's inside? 1,600 calories, 100 grams protein, 213 grams
carbohydrates, 42 grams total fat, 120 grams cholesterol, 6 grams
saturated fat, 2,490 milligrams sodium, 35 grams dietary fiber

Day 7

Breakfast
½ cup egg substitute made into an omelet filled with
¼ cup diced tomatoes,
¼ cup diced green pepper, and
1 cup sautéed spinach and topped with
1 slice soy cheese
1 cup calcium-fortified orange juice
Herbal tea

Midmorning Snack
1 Carrot Flax Muffin*
Herbal tea

Lunch
1 serving Hummus and Tzatziki Wrap*
½ cup tabbouleh
5 pitted Kalamata olives

Midafternoon Snack
6 ounces nonfat yogurt

Dinner
1 serving Pepper Mustard Chicken with Herb Sauce*
½ cup wild rice

1½ cups steamed asparagus topped with
1 teaspoon olive oil

Veg Out! *Try our Stuffed Bell Peppers as a one-pot meal that delivers a spectrum of phytonutrients and 5½ servings of veggies!*

SNACK
1 cup low-fat vanilla frozen yogurt topped with
2 tablespoons crushed walnuts and
2 tablespoons nonfat whipped topping
Herbal tea

What's inside? 1,570 calories, 92 grams protein, 212 grams carbohydrates, 40 grams total fat, 90 milligrams cholesterol, 7 grams saturated fat, 2,250 milligrams sodium, 25 grams dietary fiber

---

My Meal Plans: 2,000 Calories

This plan is typically suitable for those seeking to maintain their weight. Again, we emphasize, please consult your physician.

Day 1

BREAKFAST
¾ cup old-fashioned oats (prepared according to directions with
    water) topped with
1 cup fresh blueberries,
¼ cup nonfat plain yogurt, and
2 tablespoons ground walnuts
Black tea with ½ teaspoon cinnamon

MIDMORNING SNACK
6 ounces nonfat light yogurt topped with
¼ cup whole-grain crunchy cereal
Herbal tea

LUNCH
3 ounces chicken breast, grilled
3 cups fresh baby spinach combined with
¼ cup sliced red onion,
¼ cup sliced mushrooms,
4 cherry tomatoes, and
2 tablespoons light vinaigrette dressing
1 sprouted grain roll topped with
2 teaspoons trans fat–free light margarine

MIDAFTERNOON SNACK
1 medium apple with ½ teaspoon cinnamon
1½ ounces part-skim mozzarella cheese
Mint tea

DINNER
2 servings Vegetarian Chili* topped with
¼ cup 2 percent fat shredded cheddar cheese and
2 tablespoons light sour cream
2 cups steamed broccoli
1 ounce whole-grain crackers

SNACK
½ cup low-fat vanilla frozen yogurt topped with
½ cup sliced fresh strawberries

What's inside? 1,930 calories, 113 grams protein, 350 grams carbohydrates, 65 grams total fat, 130 milligrams cholesterol, 18 grams saturated fat, 2,770 milligrams sodium, 51 grams dietary fiber

Day 2

BREAKFAST
2 Kashi Go Lean frozen waffles topped with
2 tablespoons sugar-free syrup,
2 teaspoons light trans fat–free margarine, and
1 medium banana, sliced
1 1.3-ounce vegetarian sausage patty
Decaffeinated coffee

MIDMORNING SNACK
1 cup herbal tea with ½ teaspoon cinnamon
1 medium orange

LUNCH
Homemade "pizza": in toaster oven, heat one small whole-wheat
   pita topped with 2 ounces marinara sauce, 3 ounces sliced
   chicken, 2 ounces part-skim mozzarella cheese, and 1 cup
   sliced red, yellow, and green peppers
2 tablespoons light ranch dressing to dip
1 cup skim milk

MIDAFTERNOON SNACK
6 ounces nonfat light fruit yogurt
Low-sodium mineral water

DINNER
1 serving Mussels Fra Diavolo*
1 cup cooked brown rice
1 cup steamed broccoli topped with
1 tablespoon grated Parmesan cheese
1 cup mixed berries

Veg Out! *Try our Spinach Lasagna for a meatless meal with Italian appeal.*

SNACK
¼ cup unsalted soy nuts
2 tablespoons unsweetened dried cranberries
Decaffeinated green tea with ½ teaspoon cinnamon

What's inside? 1,960 calories, 120 grams protein, 264 grams carbohydrates, 59 grams total fat, 12 grams saturated fat, 155 milligrams cholesterol, 3,320 milligrams sodium, 34 grams dietary fiber

Day 3

BREAKFAST
1 cup shredded wheat cereal topped with
1 cup skim milk,
2 tablespoons raisins, and
½ medium banana
1 slice whole-grain toast topped with
1 tablespoon all-natural peanut butter
Decaffeinated coffee

MIDMORNING SNACK
Wedges of 1 grapefruit
Orange spice tea
6 ounces nonfat light yogurt

Lunch
1½ servings Rice, Bean, and Mango Salad*
1 small whole-wheat pita
Low-sodium sparkling water with lemon wedge

Midafternoon Snack
½ cup 1 percent cottage cheese
1 ounce dry-roasted almonds

Dinner
6 ounces baked grouper
2 cups steamed green beans
1 small sweet potato topped with
2 teaspoons trans fat–free tub margarine
Spring water

Veg Out! *Try our Summer Ratatouille for a refreshing vegetarian twist.*

Snack
5 ginger snap cookies
8 ounces chocolate soy milk

What's inside? 1,970 calories, 119 grams protein, 292 grams carbohydrates, 51 grams total fat, 95 milligrams cholesterol, 6 grams saturated fat, 1,660 milligrams sodium, 49 grams dietary fiber

Day 4

Breakfast
1 whole-wheat English muffin, toasted under broiler or in
   toaster oven, topped with
1 cup 1 percent fat cottage cheese and

¾ cup sliced strawberries and ¼ teaspoon cinnamon
1 cup coffee with nonfat creamer

MIDMORNING SNACK
2 whole-wheat graham crackers topped with
2 teaspoons almond butter
Herbal tea

LUNCH
1 large ripe tomato, cored, and stuffed with
¼ cup leftover brown rice,
3 ounces diced chicken,
2 tablespoons light mayo, and
Diced celery and onion
7 whole-grain crackers
1 medium apple

MIDAFTERNOON SNACK
1 string cheese
Decaffeinated green or black tea with lemon

DINNER
1 serving Penne with Spring Vegetables*
2 cups sliced red onion, tomato, and cucumber topped with
2 tablespoons feta cheese,
2 teaspoons olive oil, and
1 tablespoon balsamic vinegar
1 cup fresh fruit salad (blueberries, strawberries, melon) topped
    with
2 tablespoons nonfat whipped topping
Spring water

SNACK
8 ounces skim milk
Herbal tea

What's inside? 2,010 calories, 94 grams protein, 284 grams
carbohydrates, 64 grams total fat, 105 grams cholesterol, 15 grams
saturated fat, 2,900 milligrams sodium, 39 grams dietary fiber

---

Day 5

BREAKFAST
1 Mixed Berry Scone*
1 serving Chocolate and Peanut Butter Smoothie*
Decaffeinated coffee

MIDMORNING SNACK
1 medium pear
1 cup 1 percent cottage cheese

LUNCH
3 cups tossed salad greens combined with
¼ cup shredded carrots,
¼ cup sliced cucumbers,
¼ cup diced celery,
3 ounces baked barbecue flavored tofu, and
2 tablespoons light salad dressing
1 ounce whole-wheat pretzels

MIDAFTERNOON SNACK
1 cup cut-up fresh vegetables
¼ cup red pepper hummus
Herbal tea

DINNER
6 ounces roast turkey
1 small baked potato with skin topped with
¼ cup fresh salsa
2 cups steamed spinach and red peppers

Veg Out! *Enjoy our Veggie Burgers with a side of Cabbage and Apple Slaw for a picnic-perfect meal!*

SNACK
1 cup fresh diced melon
Cinnamon apple tea

What's inside? 1,990 calories, 139 grams protein, 202 grams carbohydrates 68 grams total fat, 150 milligrams cholesterol, 10 grams saturated fat, 3,700 milligrams sodium, 49 grams dietary fiber

---

Day 6

BREAKFAST
¾ cup Swiss Muesli* topped with
8 ounces (1 cup) skim milk
½ cup fresh raspberries
Green tea

MIDMORNING SNACK
1 ounce unsalted dry-roasted peanuts
2 tablespoons dried unsweetened cranberries
Herbal tea

LUNCH
1 cup Spinach Leek Soup*
2 slices cracked-wheat bread topped with

3 ounces lemon pepper turkey breast, lettuce, tomato, and
2 teaspoons Dijon mustard
1 medium apple

MIDAFTERNOON SNACK
3 cups low-fat, reduced-sodium microwave popcorn
8 ounces sparkling water with wedge of lime

DINNER
1 serving Chicken with Quinoa and Garbanzo Beans*
1½ cups tossed mixed greens topped with
¼ cup sliced radish,
¼ cup sliced carrot,
¼ cup diced celery, and
2 tablespoons balsamic vinaigrette dressing

Veg Out! *Complement our Rice, Bean, and Mango Salad with your favorite Veggie Burger for a meal in minutes!*

SNACK
1 serving Citrus Refresher*

What's inside? 2,010 calories, 113 grams protein, 280 grams carbohydrates, 55 grams total fat, 8 grams saturated fat, 135 grams cholesterol, 2,550 milligrams sodium, 44 grams dietary fiber

Day 7

BREAKFAST
½ cup egg substitute made into an omelet filled with
¼ cup diced tomatoes,
¼ cup diced green pepper, and

1 cup sautéed spinach and topped with
1 slice soy cheese
1 vegetarian breakfast sausage patty
1 cup calcium-fortified orange juice
Herbal tea

Midmorning Snack
1 Carrot Flax Muffin*
Herbal tea

Lunch
1 serving Hummus and Tzatziki Wrap*
½ cup tabbouleh
5 pitted Kalamata olives

Midafternoon Snack
1 Yogurt Parfait*
1 cup sparkling water with wedge of lime

Dinner
1 serving Pepper Mustard Chicken with Herb Sauce*
1 cup wild rice
2½ cups steamed asparagus topped with
1 teaspoon olive oil

Veg Out! *Try our Stuffed Bell Peppers as a one-pot meal that delivers a spectrum of phytonutrients and 5½ servings of veggies.*

Snack
½ cup low-fat vanilla yogurt topped with
2 teaspoons crushed walnuts and
2 tablespoons nonfat whipped topping
Herbal tea

What's inside? 1,960 calories, 119 grams protein, 268 grams carbohydrates, 58 grams total fat, 95 milligrams cholesterol, 14 grams saturated fat, 2,650 milligrams sodium, 35 grams dietary fiber

My Meal Plans: 2,400 Calories

This meal plan is for women who are either very active or who need to gain weight before becoming pregnant. Consult your physician for more individualized information.

Day 1

BREAKFAST
¾ cup old-fashioned oats (prepared with water) topped with
1 cup frozen unsweetened blueberries,
¼ cup nonfat plain yogurt,
2 tablespoons ground walnuts, and
1 tablespoon ground flaxseed
1 slice whole-wheat toast topped with
2 teaspoons light trans fat–free margarine

MIDMORNING SNACK
6 ounces nonfat light yogurt topped with
1 cup decaffeinated black tea with ½ teaspoon cinnamon or cinnamon apple tea

LUNCH
3 ounces light tuna canned in water, drained
3 cups fresh baby spinach combined with
¼ cup sliced red onion,

¼ cup sliced mushrooms,
4 cherry tomatoes,
¼ cup part-skim mozzarella cheese, and
2 tablespoons light vinaigrette dressing
1 sprouted grain roll
1 medium apple

MIDAFTERNOON SNACK
1 medium pear
¼ cup trail mix
Cinnamon apple tea

DINNER
2 servings Vegetarian Chili* topped with
¼ cup 2 percent fat shredded cheddar cheese and
2 tablespoons light sour cream
2 cups steamed broccoli
1½ ounces whole-grain crackers

SNACK
1 cup low-fat vanilla frozen yogurt
1 cup sliced strawberries
Herbal tea

What's inside? 2,340 calories, 117 grams protein, 323 grams carbohydrates, 80 grams total fat, 19 grams saturated fat, 85 milligrams cholesterol, 3,380 milligrams sodium, 60 grams dietary fiber

Day 2

BREAKFAST
2 Kashi Go Lean frozen waffles topped with
1 medium banana, sliced,
2 tablespoons sugar-free syrup, and
2 teaspoons light trans fat–free margarine
2 2-ounce vegetarian sausage patties
Decaffeinated coffee

MIDMORNING SNACK
1 cup herbal tea with ½ teaspoon cinnamon
¼ cup trail mix
1 medium orange

LUNCH
Homemade "pizza": in toaster oven, heat one small whole-wheat
    pita topped with 2 ounces marinara sauce, 3 ounces sliced
    chicken, 2 ounces part-skim mozzarella cheese, and 1 cup
    sliced red, yellow, and green peppers
2 tablespoons light ranch dressing to dip
1 cup skim milk

MIDAFTERNOON SNACK
6 ounces nonfat light fruit yogurt
Cinnamon apple tea (herbal)

DINNER
1 serving Mussels Fra Diavolo*
1 cup cooked brown rice
2 cups steamed broccoli topped with
1 tablespoon grated Parmesan cheese
1 cup mixed berries

Veg Out! *Try our Spinach Lasagna for a meatless meal with Italian appeal.*

SNACK
¼ cup unsalted soy nuts
2 tablespoons unsweetened dried cranberries
Decaffeinated green tea with ½ teaspoon cinnamon

What's inside? 2,410 calories, 148 grams protein, 321 grams carbohydrates, 67 grams total fat, 15 grams saturated fat, 160 milligrams cholesterol, 3,320 milligrams sodium, 52 grams dietary fiber

---

Day 3

BREAKFAST
1 cup shredded wheat cereal topped with
1 cup skim milk,
2 tablespoons raisins, and
½ medium banana
2 slices whole-grain toast topped with
2 tablespoons all-natural peanut butter
Decaffeinated coffee

MIDMORNING SNACK
Wedges of 1 grapefruit
Orange spice tea
6 ounces light nonfat yogurt

LUNCH
2 servings Rice, Bean, and Mango Salad*
1 small whole-wheat pita
Low-sodium sparkling water with lemon wedge

MIDAFTERNOON SNACK
1 ounce dry-roasted almonds
1 cup 1 percent fat cottage cheese

DINNER
6 ounces baked grouper
2 cups steamed green beans
1 medium sweet potato topped with
2 teaspoons trans fat–free tub margarine
1 cup melon wedges topped with
2 tablespoons light whipped cream

Veg Out! *Try our Summer Ratatouille for a refreshing vegetarian twist.*

SNACK
5 ginger snap cookies
8 ounces chocolate soy milk

What's inside? 2,370 calories, 142 grams protein, 329 grams carbohydrates, 71 grams total fat, 13 grams saturated fat, 130 milligrams cholesterol, 2,330 milligrams sodium, 54 grams dietary fiber

Day 4

BREAKFAST
1 whole-wheat English muffin, toasted under broiler or in
   toaster oven, topped with
1 cup 1 percent fat cottage cheese,
¾ cup sliced strawberries, and
¼ teaspoon cinnamon
Decaffeinated coffee with nonfat creamer

MIDMORNING SNACK
2 whole-wheat graham crackers topped with
1 tablespoon all-natural almond butter
1 tablespoon raisins
Herbal tea

LUNCH
1 large red ripe tomato stuffed with
¼ cup brown rice,
3 ounces diced chicken,
2 tablespoons light mayonnaise,
4 tablespoons diced celery and onion, and
½ cup brown rice
7 reduced-fat, woven-wheat crackers
1 medium apple

MIDAFTERNOON SNACK
1 string cheese
4 medium celery stalks
Decaffeinated green or black tea

DINNER
1 serving Penne with Spring Vegetables*
2 cups sliced red onion, tomato, and cucumber topped with
2 tablespoons feta cheese,
2 teaspoons olive oil, and
1 tablespoon balsamic vinegar
1 slice crusty whole-wheat bread topped with
2 teaspoons light trans fat–free margarine
1 cup fresh fruit salad (blueberries, strawberries, melon) topped
   with
2 tablespoons nonfat whipped topping

SNACK
8 ounces skim milk
Herbal tea

What's inside? 2,400 calories, 107 grams protein, 352 grams
carbohydrates, 75 grams total fat, 17 grams saturated fat, 110 grams
cholesterol, 3,700 milligrams sodium, 50 grams dietary fiber

Day 5

BREAKFAST
1 Mixed Berry Scone*
1 serving Chocolate and Peanut Butter Smoothie* mixed with
1 tablespoon ground flaxseed
Decaffeinated coffee

MIDMORNING SNACK
1 medium pear
1 cup 1 percent cottage cheese
Herbal tea

LUNCH
3 cups tossed salad greens topped with
¼ cup shredded carrots,
¼ cup sliced cucumbers,
¼ cup diced celery,
4 ounces baked barbecue flavored tofu, and
2 tablespoons light salad dressing
1 ounce whole-wheat pretzels

MIDAFTERNOON SNACK
1 cup cut-up fresh vegetables
¼ cup red pepper hummus
6 whole-wheat, trans fat–free crackers

DINNER
6 ounces roasted turkey
1 medium baked potato with skin, topped with
¼ cup salsa and
2 tablespoons light sour cream
2 cups spinach and peppers sautéed in
1 tablespoon olive oil and 2 cloves garlic

Veg Out! *Enjoy our Veggie Burgers with a side of Cabbage and Apple Slaw for a picnic-perfect meal!*

SNACK
½ cup nonfat vanilla pudding topped with
½ cup fresh blueberries
4 trans fat–free vanilla wafers
Cinnamon apple tea (herbal)

What's inside? 2,410 calories, 152 grams protein, 245 grams carbohydrates, 91 grams total fat, 17 grams saturated fat, 170 milligrams cholesterol, 4,100 milligrams sodium, 46 grams dietary fiber

---

Day 6

BREAKFAST
¾ cup Swiss Muesli* mixed with
8 ounces skim milk and
½ cup fresh raspberries
Decaffeinated green tea

MIDMORNING SNACK
1 ounce unsalted dry-roasted peanuts
2 tablespoons dried cranberries
Herbal tea

LUNCH
2 cups Spinach Leek Soup*
2 slices cracked-wheat bread topped with
3 ounces lemon pepper turkey breast, lettuce, and tomato, and
2 teaspoons Dijon mustard
1 medium apple with ½ teaspoon cinnamon

MIDAFTERNOON SNACK
1 crunchy trans fat–free granola bar (2 grams or more fiber, less
   than 15 grams sugar)
8 ounces almond milk

DINNER
1 serving Chicken with Quinoa and Garbanzo Beans*
1½ cups tossed mixed greens combined with
¼ cup sliced radish,
¼ cup sliced carrots,
¼ cup diced celery,
2 tablespoons balsamic vinaigrette dressing

Veg Out! *Complement our Rice, Bean, and Mango Salad with your
favorite Veggie Burger for a meal in minutes!*

SNACK
1 serving Chilled Watermelon Soup*

What's inside? 2,410 calories, 116 grams protein, 361 grams
carbohydrates, 64 grams total fat, 9 grams saturated fat, 135
milligrams cholesterol, 3,000 milligrams sodium, 44 grams dietary fiber

Day 7

BREAKFAST
½ cup egg substitute made into an omelet filled with
¼ cup diced tomato,
¼ cup diced green pepper, and
1 cup sautéed spinach and topped with
1 slice soy cheese
1 vegetarian breakfast sausage patty
1 cup calcium-fortified orange juice
1 whole-wheat English muffin
2 teaspoons trans fat–free light margarine
Herbal tea

MIDMORNING SNACK
6 ounces light fruit yogurt topped with ¼ cup low-fat granola
Herbal tea

LUNCH
1 serving Hummus and Tzatziki Wrap*
½ cup tabbouleh
5 pitted Kalamata olives
1 medium apple

MIDAFTERNOON SNACK
1½ cups fresh cut veggies (cucumber, celery, carrots, zucchini)
    dipped in
2 tablespoons light ranch dressing
6 reduced-fat, woven-wheat crackers
1 cup sparkling water with wedge of lime

DINNER
1½ servings Pepper Mustard Chicken with Herb Sauce*
1 cup wild rice

2½ cups steamed asparagus topped with
2 teaspoons olive oil
1 small cracked-wheat roll

Veg Out! *Try our Stuffed Bell Peppers as a one-pot meal that delivers a spectrum of phytonutrients and 5½ servings of veggies!*

SNACK
1 serving Almond Berry Smoothie*
Herbal tea

What's inside? 2,360 calories, 132 grams protein, 337 grams carbohydrates, 60 grams total fat, 6 grams saturated fat, 125 milligrams cholesterol, 3,650 milligrams sodium, 54 grams dietary fiber

10

Gourmet Rx: The Recipes

Now that you've learned about the baby-boosting nutrients and the foods to be fruitful, it's time to turn up the heat, turn down the lights, and enjoy these health-enhancing delights! Here you'll find more than fifty recipes, suited for the novice chef, delivering plenty of nutritional sizzle to cook your way to better health.

Soups and Salads

Each of these delicious, phytonutrient-rich soups and salads makes a perfect accompaniment or a light meal.

Pea in the Pod Soup

Sugar-balancing legumes come together with veggies to support your pea in the pod.

2 teaspoons extra-virgin olive oil
2 cups chopped yellow onion
½ cup chopped celery
1 large clove garlic, crushed
⅛ teaspoon ground red pepper or to taste
2 13.75-ounce cans reduced-sodium chicken broth
8 ounces carrots, cleaned and peeled
1 cup dry, green split peas
1 bay leaf
⅔ cup plain low-fat yogurt

In a large saucepan, heat oil over medium heat. Add onion and celery. Cook, stirring often, for 7 minutes. Add garlic and pepper. Cook, stirring, for 30 seconds. Add broth, ½ cup water, carrots, peas, and bay leaf. Bring to a boil, reduce heat, cover, and simmer until peas are tender, about 1 hour. Remove from heat and cool for 10 minutes. Remove carrots and bay leaf. Cool carrots slightly, chop into bite-size pieces, then set aside. In a blender or food processor, puree cooled soup in batches until smooth. Pour mixture back into saucepan and heat through. In a small bowl, whisk 1 cup hot soup into yogurt until blended. Whisk mixture back into remaining soup in saucepan and heat through. Stir in carrots and serve immediately.

Serves 8 (serving size: 1 cup)

Servings of fruits and vegetables: 1¼ vegetables; **fertility-boosting phytonutrients:** phytoestrogens, sulfides, carotenoids

Nutrition information: 90 calories, 5 grams protein, 1.5 grams total fat, no saturated fat, no cholesterol, 14 grams carbohydrates, 3 grams dietary fiber, 280 milligrams sodium

---

*M*aternity Minestrone

Minestrone means "big soup" in Italian, and this healthful soup is a perfect combination of flavors and textures to satisfy even the biggest of appetites.

1 cup dry kidney beans
1 cup dry cannellini beans
1 cup dry split peas
4 cloves garlic, crushed and divided
1 large yellow onion, diced and divided
1 28-ounce can crushed tomatoes
2 large carrots, sliced
1 cup broccoli florets
½ tablespoon chopped fresh basil
½ tablespoon chopped fresh oregano
½ cup uncooked small-shaped, whole-grain pasta
Freshly ground black pepper to taste

Add 6 cups water to a large pot and bring to a boil. Add the dry beans: kidney beans, cannellini beans, and peas. Add two of the chopped garlic cloves and one-half of diced onion. Simmer for 1 hour (beans should be firm and intact). Add tomatoes, carrots, broccoli, remaining onion and garlic, basil, and oregano. Simmer over medium-low heat for 20 minutes. Add pasta, cook for 10 minutes, remove from heat and serve with freshly ground pepper.

Serves 8 (serving size: 1 cup)

Servings of fruits and vegetables: 1¼ vegetables; **fertility-boosting phytonutrients:** phytoestrogens, lycopene, allicin, sulfides, carotenoids

Nutrition information: 160 calories, 9 grams protein, 0.5 gram total fat, no saturated fat, no cholesterol, 30 grams carbohydrates, 9 grams dietary fiber, 150 milligrams sodium

---

Spinach Leek Soup

With folate and sulfides, fill your bowl with this healthy delight.

2 cups vegetable or chicken broth
1 28-ounce can whole tomatoes
2 leeks, white and light green parts only, sliced
1 cup chopped carrots
2 cups fresh baby spinach
2 garlic cloves, crushed
⅓ cup fresh rosemary
Shaved Romano cheese (optional)

Simmer broth and 1½ cups water over medium heat. Add tomatoes, leeks, and carrots; cook for 15 minutes. Add spinach, garlic, and rosemary; simmer for 15 minutes. Top with Romano cheese if desired and serve.

Serves 8 (serving size: 1 cup)

Servings of fruits and vegetables: 2 vegetables; **fertility-boosting phytonutrients:** sulfides, lycopene, carotenoids

Nutrition information: 60 calories, 2 grams protein, 1 gram total fat, no saturated fat, no cholesterol, 11 grams carbohydrates, 2 grams dietary fiber, 290 milligrams sodium

Creamy Butternut Squash Soup

A warming soup boasting antioxidant carotenoids. Delicious served with a hearty whole-grain roll. Talk with your doctor about consuming soy products before or during pregnancy.

1 tablespoon extra-virgin olive oil
2 cups finely chopped yellow onions
2 cups vegetable broth
2 large butternut squash, peeled, seeded, and cubed
1 apple, peeled, cored, and diced
1 tablespoon grated gingerroot
2 cups soy milk

Add oil to a 5-quart saucepan and heat over medium heat. Add onions and cook for 15 minutes, stirring often. Add vegetable broth, squash, and apple. Bring to a boil and reduce heat to medium low. Simmer for 20 minutes. Pour 1½ cups of the soup into a blender or food processor; add grated ginger and soy milk. Puree and return to saucepan and heat through.

Serves 8 (serving size: 1 cup)

Servings of fruits and vegetables: 1 vegetable, ¼ fruit; **fertility-boosting phytonutrients:** gingerols, phytoestrogens, sulfides, quercetin, carotenoids

Nutrition information: 170 calories, 5 grams protein, 3.5 grams total fat, no saturated fat, no cholesterol, 34 grams carbohydrates, 8 grams dietary fiber, 160 milligrams sodium

Radicchio Cups with Tabbouleh

Radicchio cradles whole grains and veggies for a maternal delight.

        1 cup bulgur wheat
        3 tablespoons extra-virgin olive oil
        Juice of 1 lemon or more to taste
        Sea salt (optional)
        Freshly ground black pepper
        4 spring onions, chopped
        1 tablespoon chopped Italian flat-leaf parsley, plus
            additional sprigs for garnish
        4 tablespoons chopped fresh mint
        3 tomatoes, peeled, seeded, and diced
        ½ cup cubed low-fat mozzarella cheese
        1 head radicchio

Place the bulgur wheat in a bowl, add enough cold water to cover, and soak for 1 hour. Drain thoroughly in a sieve, pressing out the excess water. Mix together the oil, lemon juice, salt (if using), and pepper in a bowl. Add the bulgur wheat, then mix well, making sure the grains are coated with the dressing. Leave at room temperature for about 15 minutes so the bulgur wheat can absorb some of the flavors. Stir in the spring onions, parsley, mint, and tomatoes. Separate out the leaves from the radicchio and select the best cup-shaped ones. Spoon a little of the tabbouleh into each one, topping with mozzarella cubes. Arrange on individual plates or on a serving platter and garnish with flat-leaf parsley sprigs.

Serves 4 (serving size: 2 stuffed radicchio cups)

Servings of fruits and vegetables: 1 vegetable; **fertility-boosting phytonutrients:** lycopene, quercetin

---

Nutrition information: 270 calories, 9 grams protein, 13 grams total fat, 2.5 grams saturated fat, 5 milligrams cholesterol, 33 grams carbohydrates, 8 grams dietary fiber, 95 milligrams sodium

---

Garden Garbanzo Soup

Low-GI beans star in this fresh veggie soup to keep blood sugar on an even keel and deliver free-radical fighting antioxidants.

1 tablespoon extra-virgin olive oil
1 medium yellow onion, diced
1 medium red bell pepper, chopped fine
2 cloves garlic, crushed

  4 cups chicken or vegetable broth
  2 cups broccoli florets
  3 carrots, sliced
  1 15-ounce can garbanzo beans (chickpeas), drained

In a soup pot, heat oil over medium heat. Add onion and cook until translucent. Add red bell pepper, garlic, and broth, stirring well. Add broccoli, carrots, and garbanzo beans. Simmer over medium heat for 20 minutes just until vegetables are crisp tender and beans are firm.

  Serves 6 (serving size: 1 cup)

Servings of fruits and vegetables: 2¼ vegetables; **fertility-boosting phytonutrients:** lycopene, quercetin, sulfides, phytoestrogens, carotenoids

---

Nutrition information: 170 calories, 6 grams protein, 3.5 grams total fat, no saturated fat, no cholesterol, 28 grams carbohydrates, 6 grams dietary fiber, 550 milligrams sodium

---

Green Gazpacho

Tomatillos, a fruit also known as a Mexican green tomato, steal the show in this delicious "it's great to be green" version of gazpacho!

  1 cup fat-free chicken or vegetable broth
  1 28-ounce can tomatillos, drained
  1 medium cucumber, peeled, seeded, and chopped
  ½ cup packed baby spinach leaves
  12 cups packed torn romaine or other dark green lettuce

½ medium green bell pepper, seeded and chopped
½ medium white onion, chopped
2 tablespoons chopped fresh cilantro leaves
2 cloves garlic, chopped
1 tablespoon canned diced green chilies
1 tablespoon extra-virgin olive oil
Juice of 1 lime or to taste
¼ teaspoon cumin powder

Place broth, tomatillos, cucumber, spinach, lettuce, green pepper, onion, cilantro, garlic, and green chilies in blender and puree until smooth. Add oil, lime juice, and cumin. Puree again until smooth. Transfer to bowl or pitcher and chill.

Serves 8 (serving size: 1 cup)

Servings of fruits and vegetables: 2 vegetables; **fertility-boosting phytonutrients:** carotenoids, sulfides, phytoestrogens

Nutrition information: 70 calories, 3 grams protein, 3 grams total fat, no saturated fat, no cholesterol, 11 grams carbohydrates, 3 grams dietary fiber, 65 milligrams sodium

Rice, Bean, and Mango Salad

A tropical treat that combines carotenoids, whole grains, and legumes for baby-boosting balanced nutrition.

2 cups cooked brown rice
1 15-ounce can red kidney beans, drained and rinsed
¾ cup finely chopped green bell pepper

½ cup fresh mango, cut in ½-inch pieces
½ cup finely chopped red onion
½ cup well-drained salsa
Sea salt and freshly ground pepper to taste
2 tablespoons chopped fresh cilantro

In a large bowl, combine rice, beans, bell pepper, mango, and onion. Add salsa and mix into salad. Season to taste with sea salt and pepper. Sprinkle with cilantro and serve.

Serves 8 (serving size: 1 cup)

Servings of fruits and vegetables: ½ vegetable; **fertility-boosting phytonutrients:** carotenoids, lycopene, sulfides, phytoestrogens

Nutrition information: 140 calories, 5 grams protein, 0.5 gram total fat, no saturated fat, no cholesterol, 27 grams carbohydrates, 7 grams dietary fiber, 105 milligrams sodium

Watercress, Green Bean, and Radish Salad

A crunchy and refreshing salad with a tangy bite, this dish delivers fiber, folate, and sulfide compounds to protect against free radical damage.

1 pound fresh green beans, trimmed
¼ cup fresh lemon juice
2 teaspoons Dijon mustard
2 tablespoons white wine vinegar
3 tablespoons extra-virgin olive oil

½ cup vegetable broth
1 cup chopped watercress leaves
1 bunch watercress ends, trimmed
2 cups thinly sliced radish

Cook beans in boiling water for 5 minutes. Drain and pat dry. In a medium bowl, whisk lemon juice, mustard, vinegar, oil, and broth. Add watercress leaves. Toss beans, trimmed watercress leaves, and radish with dressing in a bowl.

Serves 4 (serving size: 1 cup)

Servings of fruits and vegetables: 2 vegetables; **fertility-boosting phytonutrients:** carotenoids, sulfides

---

Nutrition information: 150 calories, 3 grams protein, 11 grams total fat, 1.5 grams saturated fat, no cholesterol, 13 grams carbohydrates, 5 grams dietary fiber, 160 milligrams sodium

---

Cabbage and Apple Slaw

Full of fiber, this crisp slaw may help to reduce inflammation and free radicals.

3 apples, cored and sliced thin
Juice of 1 lemon
2 cups thinly sliced red cabbage
½ cup raisins
⅓ cup walnuts
⅓ cup low-fat plain yogurt

1 teaspoon grated fresh gingerroot
½ teaspoon ground cinnamon
½ teaspoon honey

Cover apples with lemon juice to prevent browning. Combine apples, cabbage, raisins, and walnuts in a bowl. Whisk together yogurt, gingerroot, cinnamon, and honey in another small bowl. Pour dressing over slaw, chill, and serve.

Serves 4 (serving size: 1 cup)

Servings of fruits and vegetables: 2 fruits, ½ vegetable; **fertility-boosting phytonutrients:** gingerols, quercetin, sulfides

Nutrition information: 200 calories, 5 grams protein, 6 grams total fat, no saturated fat, no cholesterol, 36 grams carbohydrates, 5 grams dietary fiber, 25 milligrams sodium

Fish and Seafood

These delicious fish dishes provide baby-boosting B vitamins and omega-3 fatty acids.

Salmon Burgers

These quick and easy burgers are full of omega-3 fatty acids to balance blood sugar and boost fertility with the added benefit of calcium for strong bones and teeth for your baby.

1 slice whole-grain bread, toasted and crumbled
⅓ cup wheat germ
1 16-ounce can Atlantic pink salmon, drained
2 egg whites
½ cup chopped onion
Vegetable oil spray
Freshly ground black pepper, to taste

Preheat oven to 350°F. Mix the toasted crumbs with wheat germ. Mix drained salmon, egg whites, and onion into breadcrumb mixture. Form four patties. Refrigerate, covered. Spray an ovenproof skillet to coat with vegetable oil and heat to medium. Cook salmon patties approximately 5 minutes each side. Transfer skillet to preheated oven and bake 20 minutes. Top with freshly ground black pepper.

Serves 4 (serving size: 1 salmon burger)

Servings of fruits and vegetables: ¼ vegetable; **fertility-boosting phytonutrients:** phytoestrogens, quercetin

Nutrition information: 240 calories, 29 grams protein, 10 grams total
fat, 2 grams saturated fat, 50 milligrams cholesterol, 10 grams
carbohydrates, 2 grams dietary fiber, 680 milligrams sodium

Sautéed Cod with Lentils

*With selenium-rich cod and fiber- and phytoestrogen-rich lentils, this
fish dish may help to prevent gestational diabetes and reduce inflammatory factors that hamper fertility.*

1 cup dry lentils
2 tablespoons extra-virgin olive oil
1 cup finely chopped yellow onion
2 large garlic cloves, chopped
1¼ teaspoons sea salt (optional)
1 tablespoon fresh lemon juice
¼ teaspoon plus ⅛ teaspoon freshly ground black pepper
4 5- to 6-ounce pieces cod fillet, ¾ to 1 inch thick
Vegetable oil spray
Lemon wedges for garnish

Cover lentils with cold water by 1½ inches in a 2-quart
saucepan and bring to a boil. Simmer, uncovered, until lentils are
just tender, about 25 minutes. Drain in a sieve set over a bowl,
reserving ½ cup cooking liquid.

While lentils are simmering, add olive oil to a 2- to 3-quart
saucepan over medium-low heat, then stir in onion, garlic, and ¾
teaspoon salt (if using) and cook, covered, stirring occasionally,
until pale golden, about 10 minutes. Remove lid and cook, uncovered, stirring occasionally, until golden, 5 to 10 minutes more.
Stir in lentils and enough reserved cooking liquid to moisten (¼
to ½ cup); cook until heated through. Just before serving, stir in

lemon juice and ¼ teaspoon pepper. While the onion finishes cooking, pat cod dry and sprinkle with remaining salt (if using) and pepper. Spray a 10- to 12-inch nonstick skillet; heat skillet over medium-high heat, then sauté fish, turning once, until browned and just cooked through, 6 to 8 minutes total. Serve fish with lentils.

Serves 4 (serving size: 1 cod fillet plus ½ cup lentils)

Servings of fruits and vegetables: 1 vegetable; **fertility-boosting phytonutrients:** quercetin, phytoestrogens, allicin

Nutrition information: 380 calories, 44 grams protein, 8 grams total fat, 1 gram saturated fat, 75 milligrams cholesterol, 32 grams carbohydrates, 15 grams dietary fiber, 530 milligrams sodium

Moroccan Fish Tagine

A fish medley sure to please, this recipe provides a spectrum of antioxidants, B vitamins, omega-3 fatty acids, and other baby-boosting nutrients in one simple dish.

¼ cup finely chopped cilantro
2 teaspoons sweet paprika
1 teaspoon ground ginger
8 saffron threads or ¼ teaspoon ground turmeric
Pinch cayenne or other hot ground pepper
Juice of ½ lemon
2 tablespoons extra-virgin olive oil
24 ounces cod or other firm white fish cut in 4 pieces
4 cups seeded and chopped fresh tomatoes, preferably plum
   tomatoes

2 garlic cloves, chopped fine
1 teaspoon ground cumin
¼ teaspoon salt
2 medium carrots, peeled and cut in ¾-inch slices
1 15-ounce can garbanzo beans, drained and rinsed
1 large yellow onion, sliced thin
1 lemon, peeled, sliced thin, and seeded
8 large green pitted olives, such as Sicilian-style
Finely chopped cilantro for garnish

In medium bowl, combine cilantro, paprika, ginger, saffron or turmeric, hot pepper, and fresh lemon juice. Mix in olive oil. Add fish, turning to coat well. Cover and marinate in refrigerator for 1 to 8 hours, turning fish once. Place tomatoes, garlic, cumin, and salt in large saucepan over medium-high heat. Cook, stirring occasionally, until tomatoes are soft for 4 to 8 minutes, reducing heat to medium low if necessary. Place sauce in a 10-inch sauté pan and arrange carrots to cover bottom. Layer garbanzo beans over carrots, then onions on top. Spread tomato sauce over onions. Cover and cook over medium-high heat for 10 minutes. Remove fish from marinade and place over tomato sauce. Arrange lemon slices over fish, spooning some of the marinade over lemons. Add olives. Cover and cook until fish is opaque throughout and flakes easily, about 10 minutes. Using slotted spoon, carefully remove fish and set aside. Divide rest of tagine among four plates. Set fish on top. Sprinkle cilantro for garnish.

Serves 4 (serving size: 6 ounces fish with ¼ of veggie and bean mixture)

Servings of fruits and vegetables: 2½ vegetables; **fertility-boosting phytonutrients:** gingerols, sulfides, curcumin, quercetin, lycopene, phytoestrogens

Nutrition information: 450 calories, 45 grams protein, 12 grams total fat, 1.5 grams saturated fat, 80 milligrams cholesterol, 39 grams carbohydrates, 8 grams dietary fiber, 610 milligrams sodium

Walnut-Encrusted Trout over Japonica Rice with Bell Peppers

A simple dish providing omega-3 fatty acids, vitamin B$_6$, plus whole grains and antioxidant lycopene, in just 30 minutes you'll have a gourmet meal, full of heal appeal.

⅛ cup walnuts, crushed
2 egg whites
½ cup Black Japonica rice (preferably Lundberg)
1 medium red bell pepper, diced
1 cup chopped onion
4 teaspoons extra-virgin olive oil
2 6-ounce trout fillets (or 1 12-ounce fillet cut into two pieces)

Place walnuts on a plate. Add egg whites to a shallow bowl. Bring 2 cups of water to a boil in a medium saucepan, add rice, and cook according to package instructions. In a skillet, sauté chopped red pepper and onion in 2 teaspoons olive oil. Remove to a plate; return to pan on burner heated to medium high and add remaining olive oil. Dip trout in egg whites, then in walnuts; place in sauté pan. Cook fillets 4 to 6 minutes per side, turning once. Reheat pepper and onion mixture. Arrange fish over rice, top with red pepper and serve.

Serves 2 (serving size: 1 trout fillet with 1 cup prepared rice and pepper mixture)

Servings of fruits and vegetables: 2 vegetables; **fertility-boosting phytonutrients:** quercetin, lycopene

Nutrition information: 520 calories, 34 grams protein, 23 grams total fat, 4 grams saturated fat, 80 milligrams cholesterol, 50 grams carbohydrates, 6 grams dietary fiber, 70 milligrams sodium

Citrus Sea Bass

Sea bass is a delicious fish that provides vitamin B$_6$ to reduce homocysteine and protect the heart. The oriental marinade also delivers flavorful phytonutrients including folate, gingerols, and vitamin E.

½ cup pineapple juice
½ cup orange juice
⅓ cup lite soy sauce
2 tablespoons peeled and finely chopped fresh gingerroot
2 tablespoons oriental sesame oil
⅛ teaspoon cayenne pepper
4 6-ounce sea bass fillets
Chopped green onions or lemongrass for garnish

Mix pineapple and orange juice, soy sauce, ginger, sesame oil, and cayenne pepper in 8-inch square glass baking dish. Add fish, turning to coat both sides. Chill for 2 hours, turning fish occasionally. Place steamer rack in large skillet and arrange fish on rack. Pour marinade into skillet under rack and bring to a boil. Cover skillet and steam fish just until opaque in center, about 8 minutes. Transfer fish to plates. Remove steamer rack from skillet. Boil marinade until reduced enough to coat spoon, about 5 minutes; spoon over fish. Top with green onions or lemongrass and serve.

Serves 4 (serving size: 1 sea bass fillet with sauce)

Servings of fruits and vegetables: none; **fertility-boosting phytonutrients:** quercetin, gingerols

Nutrition information: 270 calories, 33 grams protein, 10 grams total fat, 2 grams saturated fat, 70 milligrams cholesterol, 10 grams carbohydrates, no dietary fiber, 650 milligrams sodium

Sesame Salmon Roulades

These easy and elegant roll-ups provide a powerful punch of protein and omega-3 fatty acids plus vitamin E. Serve with brown rice and asparagus for the perfect complement.

4 3-ounce salmon fillets
2 tablespoons lite soy sauce
2 tablespoons grated fresh gingerroot
¼ cup fresh lemongrass
Juice and zest of 1 lemon
1 tablespoon oriental sesame oil
1 teaspoon crushed black peppercorns
¼ cup sesame seeds

Slice fillets horizontally to remove scales. Heat grill or grill pan. Mix soy sauce, half of the grated gingerroot, lemongrass, and lemon zest and juice; set aside. Brush fillets with oil and rub with remaining half of the grated gingerroot.

Tightly roll salmon filet and secure with toothpick. Combine peppercorns and sesame seeds in a shallow dish. Coat salmon roulade with sesame seed and black pepper mixture, spray with additional oil to coat. Arrange roulades on a piece of heavy-duty aluminum foil to form a shallow baking pan. Place on grill, cook for about 4 to 6 minutes per side. Drizzle or serve with soy mixture.

Serves 4 (serving size: 1 roulade)

Servings of fruits and vegetables: none; **fertility-boosting phytonutrients:** gingerols

Nutrition information: 280 calories, 24 grams protein, 19 grams total fat, 4 grams saturated fat, 70 milligrams cholesterol, 3 grams carbohydrates, 1 gram dietary fiber, 320 milligrams sodium

Shrimp and Asian Veggie Stir-Fry

Cast the nets and tip the scales in favor of your health and fertility! Shrimp, a low-mercury sea treat, teams up with Asian veggies for a dish that's teeming with flavor, fiber, and nutrients such as sulfides, omega-3 fats, folate, vitamin E, and gingerols.

1 pound shrimp, peeled and deveined
3 tablespoons orange juice
¼ teaspoon ground ginger
2 cloves garlic, sliced
1 tablespoon sesame seeds
2 teaspoons oriental sesame oil
2 cups sliced bok choy
1 medium red bell pepper, seeded and sliced

1 cup snow peas
½ medium yellow onion, sliced

Combine shrimp, orange juice, ginger, garlic, and sesame seeds in a large food storage bag and marinate in the refrigerator for 30 minutes. Heat a wok or a skillet to medium high. Drain shrimp and add with sesame oil to wok. Cook for 4 to 5 minutes until shrimp are opaque. Add bok choy, bell pepper, snow peas, and onion. Stir and cook about 2 minutes until vegetables are crisp tender. Serve over brown rice.

Serves 4 (serving size: ¼ pound shrimp, ½ cup brown rice, and ¼ stir-fried veggies)

Servings of fruits and vegetables: 1 vegetable; **fertility-boosting phytonutrients:** lycopene, carotenoids, allicin, gingerols, quercetin

Nutrition information: 300 calories, 29 grams protein, 6 grams total fat, 1 gram saturated fat, 220 milligrams cholesterol, 33 grams carbohydrates, 4 grams dietary fiber, 320 milligrams sodium

Mussels Fra Diavolo

*Mussels are a rich source of vitamin B_{12}, a critical nutrient in the manufacture of DNA, as well as in pernicious anemia, which is commonly experienced during pregnancy. It's also important in reducing levels of heart-harming homocysteine. **Note:** The alcohol burns off during cooking, so there is no concern relating to alcohol consumption with this dish.*

2 pounds frozen green-lipped New Zealand mussels, cleaned and debearded

2 cups white wine
4 garlic cloves, crushed
2 tablespoons extra-virgin olive oil
2 14.5-ounce cans no-salt-added diced tomatoes
1 tablespoon crushed red pepper
3 cups vegetable broth

Place mussels in a stockpot with wine, garlic, and olive oil; cover and simmer over medium-high heat. Add tomatoes, red pepper, and half of vegetable broth. Cover and simmer for 20 minutes. Add remaining vegetable broth to desired consistency. Serve with linguine.

Serves 4 (serving size: ¼ pound mussels plus sauce)

Servings of fruits and vegetables: 1½ vegetables; **fertility-boosting phytonutrients:** lycopene, lignans, allicin

Nutrition information: 390 calories, 29 grams protein, 13 grams total fat, 2 grams saturated fat, 65 milligrams cholesterol, 21 grams carbohydrates, 3 grams dietary fiber, 940 milligrams sodium

Grilled Halibut with Rosemary and Tomato-Basil Sauce

A meaty fish meal, halibut provides a plethora of protein, omega-3 fatty acids, and baby-boosting vitamins.

4 4-ounce halibut fillets
2 tablespoons fresh lemon juice
1 tablespoon plus 1 teaspoon extra-virgin olive oil

1 teaspoon crushed dried rosemary
Sea salt and freshly ground black pepper, to taste
½ cup diced ripe tomatoes
¼ cup chopped fresh basil
2 tablespoons finely chopped scallions
1 tablespoon red wine vinegar
½ teaspoon grated orange zest

Place halibut fillets in a large, shallow dish. In a small bowl, mix together lemon juice, 1 tablespoon olive oil, and rosemary. Season with salt and pepper to taste. Pour marinade over fish and turn to coat both sides. Cover and refrigerate for at least 30 minutes or for up to 4 hours. Drain fish and place on a greased grill 4 inches from the heat source and cook, turning once, until opaque throughout, about 10 minutes per inch of thickness. Meanwhile, in a small bowl whisk until well blended tomatoes, basil, scallions, vinegar, remaining olive oil, and orange zest. Season with salt and pepper to taste. Heat sauce in a small saucepan on low heat until warm. Place grilled fish on large serving platter and spoon sauce over top.

Serves 4 (serving size: 1 halibut fillet plus sauce)

Servings of fruits and vegetables: ½ vegetable; **fertility-boosting phytonutrients:** allicin, lycopene

Nutrition information: 210 calories, 31 grams protein, 8 grams total fat, 1 gram saturated fat, 45 milligrams cholesterol, 3 grams carbohydrates, less than 0.5 gram dietary fiber, 85 milligrams sodium

*F*lorida-Style Mahimahi

Fish on! In honor of the "Father of the Grill," this fish—known to some as "dolphin"—is light, satisfying, and full of protein. Serve with a simple brown rice pilaf and mixed vegetables. Voilà—tropical delight!

> 4 6-ounce mahimahi fillets
> 2 tablespoons Italian dressing (nonhydrogenated)
> Juice of 1 lemon
> Lemon wedges for garnish

Marinate mahimahi in Italian dressing and lemon juice for 30 minutes to 1 hour. Turn the grill to medium high. Place mahimahi on grill and cook for 4 to 6 minutes per side or until fish is opaque. Serve garnished with lemon wedges.

Serves 4 (serving size: 1 mahimahi fillet)

Servings of fruits and vegetables: none; **fertility-boosting phytonutrients:** none

Nutrition information: 210 calories, 40 grams protein, 3.5 grams total fat, 0.5 gram saturated fat, 160 milligrams cholesterol, 2 grams carbohydrates, no dietary fiber, 310 milligrams sodium

Garden Entrées

On the lighter side, these garden-fresh recipes provide a spectrum of antioxidant phytonutrients.

Vegetable Frittata

A delicious baked-egg dish providing protein and a spectrum of inflammation-reducing veggies, make this easy dish in one pan for a no-fuss meal.

1½ teaspoons extra-virgin olive oil
1 medium yellow onion, chopped
1 medium red bell pepper, seeded and chopped
1 medium zucchini, chopped
2 cups (packed) spinach leaves
3 large eggs
6 large egg whites
1 ounce low-fat shredded mozzarella cheese
1 cup chopped tomatoes
1 tablespoon chopped fresh basil
¼ teaspoon salt
¼ teaspoon freshly ground black pepper

Preheat broiler. Heat olive oil in 10-inch-diameter nonstick skillet over medium-high heat. Add onion and bell pepper; sauté until golden, about 8 minutes. Add zucchini; sauté until tender, about 5 minutes. Add spinach; stir until wilted, about 1 minute. Whisk eggs and egg whites in medium bowl to blend. Pour egg mixture over hot vegetables in skillet, stirring gently to combine. Reduce heat to medium low. Cook without stirring until eggs are set on bottom, about 5 minutes. Sprinkle mozzarella over egg mixture and then place under broiler. Broil until the cheese melts, about 2 minutes. Top with tomatoes, basil, salt, and pepper.

Serves 4 (serving size: ¼ of frittata)

Servings of fruits and vegetables: 1½ vegetables; **fertility-boosting phytonutrients:** lutein, lycopene, sulfides, carotenoids, quercetin

Nutrition information: 160 calories, 15 grams protein, 8 grams fat, 2.5 grams saturated fat, 185 milligrams cholesterol, 9 grams carbohydrates, 2 grams dietary fiber, 360 milligrams sodium

Vegetarian Chili

A healthy twist on a favorite comfort food, our chili uses textured vegetable protein, which can be found at a health-food store or natural grocery stores. Talk with your doctor about consuming soy products before or during pregnancy.

1 cup textured vegetable protein (TVP)
1 28-ounce can chopped tomatoes
2 15-ounce cans kidney beans
1 teaspoon red pepper flakes (optional)
1 teaspoon chili powder
3 cloves garlic, minced
1½ cups chopped onion
1 green pepper or chili pepper, diced
1 cup broccoli

Bring 1 cup water to a boil; add TVP. Stir, remove from heat, and let stand. Combine tomatoes and kidney beans in a medium pot over medium heat. Add red pepper flakes (if using) and chili powder, mixing well. Add garlic, 1 cup of the onion, pepper, and TVP, stirring well. Simmer for 15 to 20 minutes. Blanch broccoli, and add at last 5 minutes of cooking. Top with remaining chopped onions and serve.

Serves 8 (serving size: 1 cup)

Servings of fruits and vegetables: 1 ½ vegetables; **fertility-boosting phytonutrients:** lutein, lycopene, sulfides, phytoestrogens, carotenoids

---

Nutrition information: 140 calories, 9 grams protein, 1 gram fat, no saturated fat, no cholesterol, 26 grams carbohydrates, 7 grams dietary fiber, 500 milligrams sodium

---

*H*ummus and Tzatziki Wrap

A Greek treat, this simple fare will help you keep your health under wraps with its low-GI whole grains, phytoestrogens, and vitamin E.

1 15-ounce can garbanzo beans, drained
2 cloves garlic, crushed
1 tablespoon tahini (sesame paste)
2 cucumbers, peeled and chopped
2 cups plain nonfat yogurt
4 whole-wheat pitas
4 large slices of tomato

In a food processor, add garbanzo beans, garlic, tahini, and ¼ cup water. Process until smooth. In a small bowl, mix together the cucumbers and yogurt. Spread hummus on pita and top with yogurt and cucumber mixture and a tomato slice.

Serves 2 (serving size: 1 pita sandwich)

Servings of fruits and vegetables: 1 vegetable; **fertility-boosting phytonutrients:** allicin, phytoestrogens

Nutrition information: 300 calories, 15 grams protein, 4 grams total fat, 0.5 gram saturated fat, 5 milligrams cholesterol, 54 grams carbohydrates, 8 grams dietary fiber, 540 milligrams sodium

*A*sparagus, Mushroom, and Tomato Melt

A melt-in-your mouth delight, full of phyte, this veggie-full sandwich is toasty and satisfying. Talk with your doctor about consuming soy products before or during pregnancy.

2 4-inch-round whole-wheat pitas
2 cups asparagus, canned or freshly sautéed
1 medium tomato, sliced
1 cup sliced mushrooms
Sweet onion slices
Freshly ground black pepper
2 slices pepper jack soy cheese

Preheat oven to 350°F. Slice pitas in half. Layer asparagus, tomato, mushrooms, and onion (as many slices as desired) in pita. Grind black pepper, top with a slice of soy cheese, and bake for 15 minutes.

Serves 2 (serving size: 1 pita)

Servings of fruits and vegetables: 3 vegetables; **fertility-boosting phytonutrients:** lycopene, phytoestrogens

Nutrition information: 180 calories, 13 grams protein, 3.5 grams total fat, no saturated fat, no cholesterol, 29 grams carbohydrates, 7 grams dietary fiber, 410 milligrams sodium

Penne with Spring Vegetables

This light, satisfying, and colorful pasta dish boasts good carbs and fats plus a bevy of phytonutrients.

1 pound dried penne (whole-wheat, spelt, or quinoa)
2 tablespoons extra-virgin olive oil
6 cloves garlic, chopped
1 medium yellow onion, chopped fine
2 large orange bell peppers, seeded and cut into ¼-inch-thick strips
1 large yellow summer squash, halved, seeded, and sliced thin
2 large tomatoes, peeled, seeded, and chopped
1 cup sliced oil-cured black olives
1 tablespoon balsamic vinegar
1 teaspoon sea salt, optional
⅓ cup sliced basil
¼ cup grated Parmesan cheese

Cook penne according to package directions.

Meanwhile, in a large saucepan, heat oil over medium-high heat. Add garlic and onion and cook for 3 minutes. Stir in peppers and squash, cooking for about 5 minutes, until tender.

Reduce heat to medium; add tomato, olives, vinegar, and salt. Cook for 4 to 5 minutes. Gently stir in penne and toss in basil. Serve with grated cheese.

Serves 6 (serving size: ⅙ of pasta and vegetables)

Servings of fruits and vegetables: 2 vegetables; **fertility-boosting phytonutrients:** lycopene, sulfides

Nutrition information: 400 calories, 15 grams protein, 10 grams total fat, 2 grams saturated fat, 5 milligrams cholesterol, 70 grams carbohydrates, 13 grams dietary fiber, 260 milligrams sodium

Spinach Lasagna

Layer on the protection! Our lasagna combines phytoestrogen-rich tofu with full-of-folate spinach for taste and health. Talk with your doctor about consuming soy products before or during pregnancy.

2 tablespoons extra-virgin olive oil
1 cup minced shallots
1 bunch spinach, cleaned and chopped
1 teaspoon ground nutmeg
12 whole-wheat lasagna noodle strips, cooked al dente (slightly undercooked) and drained
6 cups no-salt-added tomato sauce
1 cup mashed firm tofu
½ cup reduced-fat shredded mozzarella cheese
Pinch sea salt
Freshly ground black pepper to taste

Preheat oven to 350°F. Heat oil in skillet and sauté shallots until transparent. Add spinach and nutmeg. In a large baking dish, layer lasagna strips, tomato sauce, spinach mixture, and tofu, until lasagna is used up. Season with salt and pepper. Finish with a layer of tomato sauce and top with low-fat mozzarella. Cover and bake for 20 to 30 minutes.

Serves 8 (serving size: ⅛ of lasagna)

Servings of fruits and vegetables: 4 vegetables; **fertility-boosting phytonutrients:** lycopene, sulfides, phytoestrogens

Nutrition information: 330 calories, 16 grams protein, 10 grams total fat, 1.5 grams saturated fat, 5 milligrams cholesterol, 48 grams carbohydrates, 9 grams dietary fiber, 115 milligrams sodium

Summer Ratatouille

*A slew of veggies mix and mingle for a flavor delight to reduce inflammation, balance blood sugar, and fight free radicals. **Note:** Eggplant is very porous and absorbs oil like a sponge, so it typically cooks in plenty of oil. To slash fat, cook the eggplant in a combination of chicken broth and olive oil—a chef's trick that imparts flavor while reducing fat.*

1 large eggplant (about 2 pounds)
1 teaspoon sea salt (optional)
4 teaspoons olive oil
2 medium yellow squash (8 ounces each), chopped
1 medium yellow onion, cut into thin wedges
3 tablespoons reduced-sodium chicken broth

3 large garlic cloves, minced
1 28-ounce can no-salt-added whole tomatoes
1 small fennel bulb, trimmed and chopped
2 tablespoons chopped fresh oregano
1 teaspoon chopped fresh rosemary, plus sprigs for garnish
1 medium green bell pepper, seeded and chopped

Slice eggplant crosswise. Sprinkle on both sides with ½ teaspoon salt (if using). Set on double layer of paper towels and let stand for 15 minutes. Rinse off eggplant, pat dry with clean paper towels. Cut eggplant into cubes.

Heat 2 teaspoons of the olive oil in large nonstick skillet over medium-high heat. Sauté squash and onion until onion is soft, about 5 minutes. Transfer to large bowl. Add another 1 teaspoon of the oil and broth to skillet. Stir in eggplant and reduce heat to medium. Cover and cook, stirring occasionally, until eggplant is tender, about 12 minutes.

Add to vegetables in bowl. Add remaining oil and garlic to skillet and cook for 30 seconds. Stir in tomatoes, fennel, oregano, and chopped rosemary, breaking up tomatoes with spoon. Cover and simmer for 5 minutes. Stir in green pepper. Cover and simmer for 7 minutes longer.

Return vegetables to skillet. Sprinkle with remaining salt and bring to a boil. Cook, uncovered, for 3 minutes, stirring occasionally. Serve warm or at room temperature, garnished with sprigs of rosemary.

Serves 8 (serving size: ¾ cup)

Servings of fruits and vegetables: 3 vegetables; **fertility-boosting phytonutrients:** anthocyanins, lycopene, sulfides, allicin, quercetin

---

Nutrition information: 100 calories, 4 grams protein, 3 grams total fat, no saturated fat, no cholesterol, 18 grams carbohydrates, 7 grams dietary fiber, 330 milligrams sodium

Stuffed Bell Peppers

We stuff a few simple ingredients into peppers to provide sugar-balancing phytoestrogens, fiber, whole grains, and antioxidants. Talk with your doctor about consuming soy products before or during pregnancy.

½ cup cubed firm tofu
½ cup reduced-fat ricotta cheese
1 large clove garlic, crushed
½ cup uncooked brown rice, such as Wehani or long-grain
1 cup broccoli florets
2 medium red bell peppers, stems and seeds removed
1 15-ounce can no-salt-added diced tomatoes

Preheat oven to 350°F. In a medium bowl, combine tofu and ricotta cheese; add in the garlic and refrigerate. Cook rice according to package instructions, set aside. Blanch broccoli in a small saucepan of boiling water; drain and set aside. Combine tofu mixture, rice, and broccoli. Spoon into whole peppers, pour diced tomatoes over. Bake for 30 minutes; allow to cool slightly before serving.

Serves 2 (serving size: 1 stuffed pepper)

Servings of fruits and vegetables: 5½ vegetables; **fertility-boosting phytonutrients:** lycopene, sulfides, phytoestrogens, carotenoids

Nutrition information: 370 calories, 18 grams protein, 7 grams total fat, 2.5 grams saturated fat, 15 milligrams cholesterol, 62 grams carbohydrates, 10 grams dietary fiber, 170 milligrams sodium

Enchilada Casserole

A feast of folate and satiating beans, this Mexican dish will help you achieve or maintain a healthy weight and keep things running smoothly.

1 medium bell pepper, seeded and chopped
1 large yellow onion, chopped
2 cloves garlic, minced
1 tablespoon canola oil
1 14-ounce can reduced-sodium black beans, not drained
1 14-ounce can pinto beans, not drained
1 16-ounce package frozen corn, thawed
1 28-ounce can pureed or crushed reduced-sodium
    tomatoes
1 tablespoon chili powder
½ teaspoon ground cumin
Dash of Tabasco, or to taste
Salt and freshly ground pepper to taste
12 whole-wheat tortillas
1 cup grated reduced-fat Jack cheese

Preheat oven to 350°F. In a large saucepan, sauté bell pepper, onion, and garlic in oil for five minutes. Add both types of beans, corn, tomatoes, chili powder, cumin, Tabasco, and salt and pepper if desired. Simmer over low heat for 15 minutes. Assemble casserole in a 9″ × 13″ baking dish. Cover bottom with one-third of bean mixture. Layer six tortillas on top of beans. Repeat once more, then end with bean mixture on top. Sprinkle cheese over the casserole and bake until hot and bubbly, about 30 to 40 minutes.

Serves 8 (serving size: ⅛ of casserole)

Servings of fruits and vegetables: 1½ vegetables; **fertility-boosting phytonutrients:** lycopene, sulfides, allicin, phytoestrogens

Nutrition information: 460 calories, 20 grams protein, 13 grams total fat, 4.5 grams saturated fat, 20 milligrams cholesterol, 69 grams carbohydrates, 11 grams dietary fiber, 800 milligrams sodium

Veggie Burgers

These hearty burgers offer phytoestrogens, vitamin E, and sulfides for cellular defense and delicious flavor. Talk with your doctor about consuming soy products before or during pregnancy.

1 carrot, grated
1 medium yellow onion, diced
1 clove garlic minced
2 teaspoons finely chopped scallions
2 tablespoons sesame oil
2 cups mashed firm tofu
1 tablespoon tamari
1 large egg, beaten, or ¼ cup liquid egg substitute

½ cup whole-grain bread crumbs
2 tablespoons chopped almonds
½ teaspoon dried thyme
½ teaspoon sea salt (optional)

Lightly sauté carrot, onion, garlic, and scallions in sesame oil. Transfer to bowl and mix in tofu, tamari, egg, bread crumbs, almonds, thyme, and salt (if using). Mix with wooden spoon to a pasty burger consistency, adding water if necessary. Shape into four patties and sauté in a large nonstick skillet or bake in oven on cookie sheet at 350°F for about 40 minutes or until golden brown. If desired, melt cheese on burgers and serve with choice of whole-grain buns or toast and condiments.

Serves 4 (serving size: 1 4-ounce burger)

Servings of fruits and vegetables: 1 vegetable; **fertility-boosting phytonutrients:** quercetin, allicin, lycopene, sulfides, vitamin E, phytoestrogens

Nutrition information: 240 calories, 13 grams protein, 15 grams total fat, 2.5 grams saturated fat, 55 milligrams cholesterol, 13 grams carbohydrates, 3 grams dietary fiber, 600 milligrams sodium

Chicken and Poultry

These delicious poultry dishes provide a bevy of B vitamins. Look for free-range poultry produced without hormones or antibiotics in your grocer's cold case.

Chicken with Quinoa and Garbanzo Beans

High in protein, this simple dish also boasts folate, phytoestrogens, and magnesium.

2 tablespoons extra-virgin olive oil
4 3-ounce boneless, skinless chicken breasts
1 medium yellow onion, diced
1 medium tomato, diced
2 large cloves garlic, crushed
1 cup chicken broth
Juice of 1 lemon
2 cups quinoa
1 16-ounce can garbanzo beans, drained and rinsed

Heat oil in medium nonstick skillet over medium-high heat. Add chicken and brown on both sides, turning pieces once, about 10 minutes, and transfer chicken to a plate. In the same pan sauté onion until lightly browned, about 5 minutes. Add tomato and garlic. Cook to soften tomatoes, stirring occasionally, for about 5 minutes. Return chicken to pan and add chicken broth and lemon juice. Cover pan tightly and simmer for 20 minutes. Add quinoa and garbanzo beans. Cover and cook until quinoa is firm and fluffy, about 20 minutes. Remove pan from heat; let sit, covered, for 10 minutes, until quinoa is fluffy and soft.

Serves 4 (serving size: 1 chicken breast plush ¼ quinoa and bean mixture)

Servings of fruits and vegetables: 1 vegetable; **fertility-boosting phytonutrients:** lycopene, allicin, quercetin

Nutrition information: 590 calories, 52 grams protein, 13 grams total fat, 2 grams saturated fat, 95 milligrams cholesterol, 67 grams carbohydrates, 12 grams dietary fiber, 250 milligrams sodium

Chicken with Ginger, Black Beans, and Rice

A Caribbean favorite providing whole grains and beans to balance blood sugar.

2 4-ounce free-range chicken breasts
Vegetable cooking spray
1 teaspoon turmeric
½ teaspoon crushed red pepper flakes
½ cup uncooked Wehani rice or brown rice
1 15-ounce can reduced-sodium black beans, drained and
    rinsed
1 tablespoon freshly grated gingerroot
2 tablespoons extra-virgin olive oil

Preheat oven to 350°F. Trim chicken breasts of all fat, add to a baking dish, spray lightly with oil. Combine turmeric and red pepper; rub into chicken breasts. Bake for 30 minutes or until juices run clear. Cook rice according to package directions. Heat black beans with grated gingerroot in a medium saucepan over medium-low heat. Serve black beans over rice with chicken.

Serves 2 (serving size: 1 chicken breast plus ½ rice and bean mixture)

Servings of fruits and vegetables: none; **fertility-boosting phytonutrients:** phytoestrogens, curcumin, gingerols

Nutrition information: 630 calories, 42 grams protein, 20 grams total fat, 3 grams saturated fat, 70 milligrams cholesterol, 69 grams carbohydrates, 15 grams dietary fiber, 500 milligrams sodium

Pepper Mustard Chicken with Herb Sauce

A flavorful chicken dish that's full of protein, this dish goes nicely with fettuccini or long-grain rice.

2 tablespoons extra-virgin olive oil
5 shallots, chopped
5 shiitake mushrooms, cleaned and quartered
5 teaspoons freshly ground black pepper
1 cup dry white wine
5 sprigs rosemary
5 sprigs thyme
2 cups reduced-sodium chicken broth
8 3-ounce boneless, skinless chicken breasts
¼ cup Dijon mustard
1 tablespoon mustard seeds

Heat oil in a large sauté pan over medium-high heat. Add shallots, mushrooms, and 1 teaspoon pepper; sauté until brown. Add wine and bring to a boil. Add rosemary and thyme; simmer for 5 minutes. Add broth and boil for 20 minutes until reduced to ¾ cup. Set aside. Preheat broiler, sprinkle remaining pepper over both sides of chicken breasts. Broil for 5 minutes per side, just until cooked through but not dry. Remove chicken from broiler. Combine Dijon mustard and seeds and brush onto chicken. Bring sauce back up to a simmer while whisking. Divide chicken among plates, spoon sauce over, and serve.

Serves 8 (serving size: 1 chicken breast plus ⅛ sauce)

Servings of fruits and vegetables: 1½ vegetables; **fertility-boosting phytonutrients:** phytoestrogens, sulfides

Nutrition information: 230 calories, 29 grams protein, 7 grams total fat, 1.5 grams saturated fat, 70 milligrams cholesterol, 8 grams carbohydrates, 1 gram dietary fiber, 310 milligrams sodium

Turkey Meatloaf with Spinach

A healthier version of an old standby, we sneak in added fiber from the oats and folate from the spinach.

½ cup rolled oats (not quick or instant)
2 large egg whites, beaten until frothy
1 cup seeded and chopped tomatoes
1¼ pounds lean ground turkey
1½ tablespoons ground chili powder
2 teaspoons dried oregano
1 teaspoon sea salt (optional)
¼ teaspoon freshly ground black pepper
1 10-ounce package frozen spinach, thawed and squeezed
    well to remove excess moisture

½ cup frozen, canned, or fresh corn kernels
Vegetable oil spray
¼ cup chili sauce or ketchup

Preheat oven to 375°F. In a large bowl, using a fork, mix together the oats, egg whites, and tomatoes. Blend in turkey, chili powder, oregano, salt, and pepper. Mix in spinach and corn. Pack mixture firmly into a 9″ × 5″ loaf pan that has been lightly coated with cooking oil spray. Bake uncovered for 45 minutes. Spread chili sauce or ketchup over top and continue baking until juices run clear when meatloaf is pierced with a knife or internal temperature registers 165°F. Remove from oven and let meatloaf sit at least 15 minutes before serving.

Serves 6 (serving size: 3 ounces meatloaf)

Servings of fruits and vegetables: 1 vegetable; **fertility-boosting phytonutrients:** lycopene, carotenoids

Nutrition information: 190 calories, 29 grams protein, 2.5 grams total fat, no saturated fat, 40 milligrams cholesterol, 15 grams carbohydrates, 5 grams dietary fiber, 290 milligrams sodium

Pot-au-Feu

A traditional French dish, this hearty stew is packed with protein plus antioxidant-rich veggies.

4 4-ounce boneless, skinless chicken breast halves
3 teaspoons fresh thyme
Freshly ground black pepper

4 cups reduced-sodium vegetable or chicken broth
2 large leeks, halved lengthwise, crosswise cut into 1-inch
   pieces
2 carrots, halved lengthwise, crosswise cut into 1-inch
   pieces
3 large plum tomatoes, seeded, cut into ¼-inch strips
1 bay leaf
3 garlic cloves, crushed
1 small zucchini, cut diagonally in ¼-inch slices
¼ cup chopped fresh Italian, flat-leaf parsley

Season chicken breasts with 1 teaspoon of the thyme and pepper. Heat large nonstick skillet over high heat and sear chicken for 2 minutes on each side. Transfer chicken to platter. Add broth, leeks, carrots, tomatoes, bay leaf, and garlic; simmer for 8 minutes. Return chicken to skillet and simmer for 10 minutes. Transfer chicken to platter and slice thinly. Discard bay leaf. Add zucchini and return chicken slices to pan. Combine remaining parsley and thyme, sprinkle over stew, and serve.

Serves: 4 (serving size: 1 chicken breast plus ¼ stew)

Servings of fruits and vegetables: 2½ vegetables; **fertility-boosting phytonutrients:** lycopene, sulfides, carotenoids

Nutrition information: 210 calories, 32 grams protein, 2 grams total fat, no saturated fat, 65 milligrams cholesterol, 16 grams carbohydrates, 3 grams dietary fiber, 670 milligrams sodium

Chicken with Julienned Vegetables

Chop, chop! A fast-fix microwave meal in minutes that delivers protein, vitamin B6, and carotenoids.

1½ tablespoons extra-virgin olive oil
1 cup julienned green and red bell peppers
1 cup julienned carrots
Salt and freshly ground pepper to taste
4 3-ounce skinless chicken breasts
4 sprigs fresh tarragon finely minced

In a microwave-safe baking dish that is just large enough to hold chicken breasts in a single layer, place half the vegetables, using some of each type. Sprinkle with salt and pepper to taste. Season chicken with salt and pepper and place on top of vegetables. Top with remaining vegetables. Drizzle with oil and then sprinkle with tarragon. Lightly cover dish with wax paper and microwave on high until chicken is tender but no longer pink, about 6 minutes if boneless, 8 to 10 minutes if bone-in. Add salt and pepper to taste if necessary.

Serves: 4 (serving size: 1 chicken breast plus ¼ vegetables)

Servings of fruits and vegetables: 1 vegetable; **fertility-boosting phytonutrients:** lycopene, carotenoids

Nutrition information: 160 calories, 20 grams protein, 7 grams total fat, 1 gram saturated fat, 50 milligrams cholesterol, 5 grams carbohydrates, 2 grams dietary fiber, 80 milligrams sodium

Grilled Chicken Kebabs

Get skewered! A colorful and delicious grill meal for a summer bar-becue that packs a nutritional punch.

½ cup low-fat plain yogurt
1 garlic clove, minced
1 teaspoon grated fresh gingerroot or ¼ teaspoon ground
   ginger
1 teaspoon tomato paste
1 tablespoon curry powder
Salt and freshly ground pepper to taste
12 ounces boneless, skinless chicken breast, cut into 24
   pieces
8 1-inch cubes fresh or canned pineapple
1 medium red onion, cut in 20 wedges
1 large green bell pepper, seeded and cut into 20 pieces
Canola oil cooking spray

In a medium bowl, combine yogurt, garlic, ginger, tomato paste, curry powder, and salt and pepper. Mix in chicken to coat on all sides. Cover bowl and refrigerate for 2 to 8 hours. Preheat grill or broiler. If using wooden skewers, soak in water for at least 15 minutes. Remove chicken from marinade, scraping off and discarding most of marinade. On each skewer, thread a piece of pineapple, then chicken, onion wedge, and green pepper. Repeat, minus pineapple, until each kebab contains 6 pieces of chicken, 5 onion wedges, 5 pieces of pepper, and 2 pineapple cubes, one cube at each end. To help prevent charring, spray kebabs with cooking oil spray. Cook skewers for 4 to 5 minutes, making sure they are far enough from the heat source to avoid charring. Turn and cook until chicken is opaque throughout, for about 4 more minutes.

Serves: 4 (serving size: 1 kebab)

Servings of fruits and vegetables: 1 vegetable; **fertility-boosting phytonutrients:** lycopene, carotenoids, quercetin, sulfides, curcumin

Nutrition information: 150 calories, 22 grams protein, 2 grams total fat, 0.5 gram saturated fat, 50 milligrams cholesterol, 12 grams carbohydrates, 2 grams dietary fiber, 90 milligrams sodium

Mediterranean Chicken

A one-dish, no-fuss meal that boasts vitamin B_6 and lycopene.

1 pint cherry tomatoes
2 tablespoons extra-virgin olive oil
2 tablespoons chopped fresh basil
10 Kalamata olives, halved
4 3-ounce boneless, skinless chicken breasts
Freshly ground black pepper

Preheat oven to 475°F. Combine tomatoes, 1 tablespoon oil, basil, and olives in a medium bowl. Set aside. Heat an ovenproof skillet with a lid over medium-high heat. Add remaining oil. Cook chicken for about 4 minutes on each side, turning once. Add tomato and olive mixture and cover. Place skillet in oven. Roast for about 20 minutes or until juices run clear. Serve with freshly ground black pepper.

Serves: 4 (serving size: 1 chicken breast plus ¼ vegetables)

Servings of fruits and vegetables: ½ vegetable; **fertility-boosting phytonutrients:** lycopene

Nutrition information: 200 calories, 20 grams protein, 11 grams total fat, 1.5 grams saturated fat, 50 milligrams cholesterol, 4 grams carbohydrates, 1 gram dietary fiber, 210 milligrams sodium

Roasted Cornish Hens

A lovely presentation that delivers protein, B vitamins, whole grains, and sulfides.

½ cup uncooked wild rice, rinsed well
½ cup uncooked brown rice
1 teaspoon minced fresh tarragon or ½ teaspoon dried
2 teaspoons extra-virgin olive oil
½ medium yellow onion, chopped fine
4 ounces mushrooms, sliced thin
¼ cup slivered blanched almonds
2 Cornish hens
1 cup fat-free reduced-sodium chicken broth
Salt and freshly ground black pepper to taste

In large saucepan, bring 3 cups of water or broth to boil. Add both rices and tarragon. Bring to boil, reduce heat, cover, and simmer for 45 minutes or until rice is tender. Transfer cooked rice to bowl. While rice is cooking, heat oil in nonstick pan over medium heat. Add onion and sauté until soft and translucent. Increase heat to high and add mushrooms and almonds. Sauté, stirring constantly to prevent burning, for about 3 minutes or until almonds are golden. Combine mixture with cooled rice. Preheat oven to 375°F. Rinse hens and trim excess fat; then stuff with rice mixture. Place hens on rack in shallow roasting pan, breast-side up. Roast hens, basting with broth every 15 minutes until done, about 75 minutes. (Hens are done when juices run clear when thigh is pricked with fork.) Cut each hen in half, lengthwise. Transfer any pan juices to small cup and skim off fat. Divide stuffing between four plates. Place ½ hen on top of each bed of rice. Heat pan juices in microwave, then pour over birds. Add salt and pepper to taste.

Serves: 4 (serving size: ½ hen plus ¼ rice and vegetables)

Servings of fruits and vegetables: ½ vegetable; **fertility-boosting phytonutrients:** sulfides, quercetin

Nutrition information: 380 calories, 32 grams protein, 12 grams total fat, 2 grams saturated fat, 110 milligrams cholesterol, 37 grams carbohydrates, 3 grams dietary fiber, 200 milligrams sodium

Turkey and Rice Soup

A quick and comforting soup, delivering protein and vitamin B_6.

1 tablespoon extra-virgin olive oil
1 cup diced yellow onion
½ cup sliced celery
½ cup sliced carrots
1 pound fresh skinless turkey breast, diced
2 cups vegetable broth
1 cup quick-cooking brown rice

Heat a soup pot over medium heat. Add oil and sauté onion for 1 minute. Add celery and carrots, and cook for about 5 minutes, stirring. Add turkey breast, vegetable broth, 2 cups of water, and rice. Bring to a boil and cook until rice is tender, about 15 to 20 minutes.

Serves: 4 (serving size: 1 cup)

Servings of fruits and vegetables: 1¼ vegetables; **fertility-boosting phytonutrients:** sulfides, carotenoids

Nutrition information: 360 calories, 32 grams protein, 6 grams total fat, 1 gram saturated fat, 70 milligrams cholesterol, 43 grams carbohydrates, 3 grams dietary fiber, 250 milligrams sodium

Desserts and Drinks

Who says dessert can't be healthy? Try our smoothies and desserts to please your palate without guilt.

Banana Bran Bread

A wholesome alternative to an old standby, our banana bread provides bunches of fiber and whole grains to balance blood sugar sweetly.

2 large eggs
2 cups whole-wheat flour
1 teaspoon baking powder
½ teaspoon salt
1½ cups bran cereal
3 large bananas, peeled and mashed
½ cup canola margarine (nonhydrogenated), softened
¾ cup evaporated cane sugar
½ cup chopped nuts, such as walnuts, almonds, or pecans

Preheat oven to 350°F. Break the eggs into a bowl and beat well. In another bowl, sift together the flour, baking powder, and salt. In a separate bowl, combine the cereal and mashed bananas; let this mixture stand for 5 minutes. Cream the canola margarine and sugar together, fold in the eggs, and then add the banana-cereal mixture. Beat well.

Stir in the flour mixture and the chopped nuts. Mix until the flour and nuts are evenly distributed through the mixture. Grease a 9″ × 5″ × 3″ loaf pan and spoon in the mixture. Place in the preheated oven. Bake the banana bread for 60 minutes. It is done when a toothpick inserted in the middle comes out clean. Remove the banana bread from the oven and allow to cool slightly. Turn out onto a wire rack to complete cooling.

Serves 15 (serving size: 1 slice)

Servings of fruits and vegetables: ½ fruit; **fertility-boosting phytonutrients:** none

Nutrition information: 210 calories, 5 grams protein, 8 grams total fat, 1 gram saturated fat, 35 milligrams cholesterol, 32 grams carbohydrates, 5 grams dietary fiber, 180 milligrams sodium

Carrot Flax Muffins

Delicious for breakfast or serve as a base for a scoop of frozen vanilla bean yogurt for dessert, these feel-good muffins deliver! Don't forget to flax your partner—omega-3 fatty acids are good for both of you!

2 eggs, or ½ cup liquid egg substitute
½ cup light-brown sugar
2 cups shredded carrot
½ cup flaxseed meal
1½ cups whole-wheat flour or soy flour
1 teaspoon baking soda
½ teaspoon salt

Preheat oven to 350°F. Grease muffin pan or arrange muffin cups. Beat eggs or egg substitute and sugar until light and thick. Fold in shredded carrot. Sift remaining dry ingredients together, and stir into carrot mixture just until blended. Pour batter into muffin pans and bake for 20 to 25 minutes, or until a cake tester inserted in the center comes out clean. Cool slightly, then remove from pan.

Serves 12 (serving size: 1 muffin)

Servings of fruits and vegetables: ½ vegetable; **fertility-boosting phytonutrients:** carotenoids, lignans

Nutrition information: 150 calories, 5 grams protein, 3.5 grams total fat, no saturated fat, no cholesterol, 25 grams carbohydrates, 5 grams dietary fiber, 240 milligrams sodium

Cranberry Walnut Squares

A bounty of great grains to stabilize blood sugar, reduce inflammation, and provide fiber team up with spices and fruits for a delicious morning treat or dessert with added benefits. Take this on a trail ride for two! You can find evaporated cane juice crystals in your local health-food store.

1 cup whole-grain cereal, such as wheat bran flakes, bran
   buds, Kashi 7 in the Morning
¾ cup rolled oats (not quick-cooking or instant)
⅓ cup whole-wheat flour
1 tablespoon ground flaxseeds
⅓ cup chopped walnuts
¾ cup dried cranberries
½ teaspoon baking soda
¼ teaspoon salt
1 teaspoon ground cinnamon
6 ounces nonfat vanilla yogurt

1 large egg
1 large egg white
⅓ cup expeller pressed canola oil
⅔ cup evaporated cane juice crystals
1 teaspoon vanilla extract

Preheat oven to 350°F. In a medium bowl, combine whole-grain cereal with rolled oats, flour, flaxseeds, walnuts, cranberries, baking soda, salt, and cinnamon. Set aside. In a food processor, add yogurt, egg, egg white, oil, cane juice crystals, and vanilla extract and process until smooth. Add liquid mixture to dry ingredients, and mix well. Pour batter into a lightly oiled 13″ × 9″ baking dish. Bake for 20 to 25 minutes, until golden brown. Cool, cut into squares and serve.

Serves 12 (Serving size: 1 square)

Servings of fruits and vegetables: ½ fruit; **fertility-boosting phytonutrients:** none

Nutrition information: 210 calories, 4 grams protein, 10 grams total fat, 1 gram saturated fat, 20 milligrams cholesterol, 29 grams carbohydrates, 2 grams dietary fiber, 130 milligrams sodium

*M*ixed Berry Scones

Berry delicious! Coffee-house style . . . but healthy! Our fiber-friendly scones provide delicious taste plus good carbs and fats. Feed one to your honey! Talk to your doctor about consuming soy products before or during pregnancy.

1 cup silken tofu
6 tablespoons soy margarine (trans fat free)
1 cup granulated fructose or evaporated cane juice crystals
1 teaspoon vanilla extract
1 cup low-fat buttermilk
2 large egg whites, or ¼ cup liquid egg substitute
1 cup Kashi Heart to Heart cereal, crushed into small
   pieces
1½ cups whole-wheat pastry flour
1 tablespoon baking powder
1 teaspoon cinnamon or nutmeg (optional)
1½ cups frozen mixed berries

Preheat oven to 350°F. Cream the tofu, soy margarine, cane juice crystals, and vanilla until fluffy. Add buttermilk and egg whites or egg substitutes and blend well. Add cereal, flour, baking powder, and cinnamon or nutmeg (if using) and fold gently until all ingredients are evenly blended together (may be a bit lumpy). Gently fold in berries, being careful not to overmix or break berries too much. Scoop a large, heaping spoonful of dough onto a well-oiled (or parchment-paper-lined) cookie sheet. Flatten scone slightly and sprinkle with additional cinnamon, if desired. Bake scones for 15 to 20 minutes or until slightly browned on edges, being careful not to overbake.

Serves 24 (serving size: 1 scone)

Servings of fruits and vegetables: none; **fertility-boosting phytonutrients:** anthocyanins, phytoestrogens

Nutrition information: 110 calories, 3 grams protein, 3.5 grams total fat, 0.5 gram saturated fat, no cholesterol, 17 grams carbohydrates, 1 gram dietary fiber, 110 milligrams sodium

Citrus Refresher

This tangy and tantalizing beverage is full of folate and antioxidants, perfect for hydrating your body and fighting the fertility foe–free radicals.

1 cup grapefruit juice
1 tablespoon fresh lime or lemon juice
1 medium orange (one slice reserved)
1 cup sparkling mineral water

Mix grapefruit juice, lime or lemon juice, and orange in a blender. Blend in high speed until mixture is combined and smooth. Pour into 2 glasses, add sparking mineral water and an orange slice.

Serves 2 (serving size: 1 cup)

Servings of fruits and vegetables: 1½ fruits; **fertility-boosting phytonutrients:** carotenoids, glutathione

Nutrition information: 90 calories, 2 grams protein, no total fat, no saturated fat, no cholesterol, 23 grams carbohydrates, 2 grams dietary fiber, no sodium

Chocolate and Peanut Butter Smoothie

Oh, yum! When biotin and folate-rich peanut butter meet mineral-rich almond milk it's a baby-boosting taste temptation.

3 tablespoons all-natural peanut butter
1½ cups chocolate almond milk
½ cup low-fat yogurt
1 cup crushed ice

Mix all ingredients in a blender on high for 2 minutes until smooth. Serve.

Serves 2 (serving size: 1 cup)

Servings of fruits and vegetables: none; **fertility-boosting phytonutrients:** phytoestrogens

Nutrition information: 280 calories, 9 grams protein, 15 grams total fat, 2 grams saturated fat, no cholesterol, 12 grams carbohydrates, 2 grams dietary fiber, 220 milligrams sodium

Yogurt Parfait

Looks gourmet, but acts healing! Layer these delicious ingredients together for a delicious dessert for two.

2 cups nonfat plain yogurt
½ cup berries, such as blueberries or raspberries (thawed if
   frozen)
¼ cup slivered almonds
1 teaspoon ground cinnamon

In a dessert bowl or wine goblet, add yogurt to dessert dish, and top with berries, almonds, and cinnamon.

Serves 2 (serving size: 1 cup)

Servings of fruits and vegetables: ¼ fruit; **fertility-boosting phytonutrients:** anthocyanins, phytoestrogens

Nutrition information: 200 calories, 13 grams protein, 7 grams total fat, 0.5 gram saturated fat, 5 milligrams cholesterol, 28 grams carbohydrates, 3 grams dietary fiber, 135 milligrams sodium

Chilled Watermelon Soup

Full of minerals and antioxidants, this chilly delight offers an abundance of health-promoting phytonutrients.

1 tablespoon chopped fresh gingerroot
½ cup light-brown sugar
Zest and juice of 2 limes or lemons
3 cups seeded and cubed watermelon

½ cup sparkling water

2 mint leaves, plus more garnish

Sauté gingerroot, brown sugar, and lemon or lime zest over medium heat for 2 minutes. Add lemon or lime juice and simmer until no liquid remains. Transfer to a blender, add watermelon, sparkling water, and mint leaves. Puree until smooth, strain into a bowl, and chill for at least 3 hours. Serve with fresh mint leaves.

Serves: 4 (serving size: 1 cup)

Servings of fruits and vegetables: ¾ fruit; **fertility-boosting phytonutrients:** lycopene, gingerols

Nutrition information: 150 calories, 1 gram protein, no total fat, no saturated fat, no cholesterol, 38 grams carbohydrates, no dietary fiber, 15 milligrams sodium

Swiss Muesli

Originally developed as a health food by a Swiss nutritionist, muesli has become a very popular breakfast cereal. Why not make your own version with this delicious recipe and sprinkle over low-fat yogurt for a healthy dessert?

1 cup halved unsalted raw cashews

3 cups rolled oats (not quick-cooking or instant)

1 cup diced dried apples

¾ cup dried currants or cranberries

½ cup toasted wheat germ

½ cup raw unsalted sunflower seeds

¼ cup raw unsalted pumpkin seeds

¼ cup evaporated cane juice crystals
1 teaspoon cinnamon

Preheat oven to 375°F. Add all ingredients to a large bowl and mix well with hands. Place in a single layer on a parchment-paper-lined cookie sheet. Bake, stirring several times, for 15 to 18 minutes, or until lightly toasted.

Serves: 12 (serving size: about ½ cup)

Servings of fruits and vegetables: 1 fruit; **fertility-boosting phytonutrients:** gingerols, anthocyanins

Nutrition information: 280 calories, 9 grams protein, 10 grams total fat, 1.5 grams saturated fat, no cholesterol, 39 grams carbohydrates, 5 grams dietary fiber, 100 milligrams sodium

---

Almond Berry Smoothie

This delicious drink provides plenty of omega-3 and vitamin E for Mom and Baby.

1 cup mixed berries, frozen
1 tablespoon flaxmeal
1 cup vanilla almond milk

Add all ingredients in a blender. Blend until smooth.

Serves: 1 (serving size: 1 cup)

Servings of fruits and vegetables: 1¼ fruits; **fertility-boosting phytonutrients:** anthocyanins, lignans

Nutrition information: 250 calories, 5 grams protein, 9 grams total fat, no saturated fat, no cholesterol, 39 grams carbohydrates, 9 grams dietary fiber, 170 milligrams sodium

Chocolate Smoothie

Have your chocolate and drink it, too! The berries, mint, and cocoa in this smoothie provide heart-healthy antioxidant phytonutrients and heavenly taste. Grab a straw and try it for dessert tonight. Talk with your doctor about consuming soy products before or during pregnancy.

¾ cup chocolate soy milk
1¼ cups frozen, unsweetened raspberries
½ medium banana, sliced
¾ cup chocolate sorbet
2 tablespoons fresh mint, chopped

Combine the soy milk, raspberries, and banana in a blender. Add the sorbet and mint. Blend until smooth.

Serves: 2 (serving size: approximately ½ cup)

Servings of fruits and vegetables: 1 fruit; **fertility-boosting phytonutrients:** phytoestrogens

Nutrition information: 200 calories, 5 grams protein, 2.5 grams total fat, no saturated fat, no trans fat, no cholesterol, 43 grams carbohydrates, 9 grams dietary fiber, 65 milligrams sodium

Appendix
Converting to Metrics

Measurement Conversions

We have included the following tables so you can easily convert measuring ingredients.

Volume Measurement Conversions	
U.S.	**Metric**
¼ teaspoon	1.25 ml
½ teaspoon	2.5 ml
¾ teaspoon	3.75 ml
1 teaspoon	5 ml
1 tablespoon	15 ml
¼ cup	62.5 ml
½ cup	125 ml
¾ cup	187.5 ml
1 cup	250 ml

Weight Conversion Measurements	
U.S.	**Metric**
1 ounce	28.4 g
8 ounces	227.5 g
16 ounces (1 pound)	455 g

Temperature Conversions

We've also included the following table and calculations so you can easily convert cooking temperatures for our recipes.

Cooking Temperature Conversions	
Celsius/Centigrade	0°C and 100°C are arbitrarily placed at the melting and boiling points of water and standard to the metric system.
Fahrenheit	Fahrenheit established 0°F as the stabilized temperature when equal amounts of ice, water, and salt are mixed.

To convert temperatures in Fahrenheit to Celsius, use this formula:

$$C = (F - 32) \times 0.5555$$

So, for example, if you are baking at 350°F and want to know that temperature in Celsius, use this calculation:

$$C = (350 - 32) \times 0.5555 = 176.66°C$$

Selected References

Chapter 1: Understanding Fertility

National Institute of Child Health and Human Development, National Institute of Health, nichd.nih.gov.

Rich-Edwards J. W., D. Spiegelman, M. Garland, E. Hertzmark, D. J. Hunter, G. A. Colditz, W. C. Willett, H. Wand, and J. E. Manson. "Physical Activity, Body Mass Index, and Ovulatory Disorder Infertility." *Epidemiology* 13 (March 2002): 184–90.

The National Women's Health Information Center, 4woman.gov.

Chapter 2: Barriers to Conception: PCOS, Insulin Resistance, and Other Hormonal Factors

Abrao, M. S., S. Podgaec, B. M. Filho, L. O. Ramos, J. A. Pinotti, and R. M. de Oliveira. "The Use of Biochemical Markers in the Diagnosis of Pelvic Endometriosis." *Human Reproduction* 12, no. 11 (November 1997): 2523–27.

Aronson, D., P. Bartha, O. Zinder, A. Kerner, E. Shitman, W. Markiewicz, G. J. Brook, and Y. Levy. "Association Between Fasting Glucose and C-Reactive Protein in Middle-Aged Subjects." *Diabetes Medicine* 21, no. 1 (January 2004): 39–44.

Bahceci, M., A. Tuzcu, N. Canoruc, Y. Tuzun, V. Kidir, and C. Aslan. "Serum C-Reactive Protein (CRP) Levels and Insulin Resistance in Non-Obese Women with Polycystic Ovarian Syndrome, and Effect of Bicalutamide on Hirsutism, CRP Levels and Insulin Resistance." *Hormone Research* 62, no. 6 (2004): 283–87.

Bajari, T. M., J. Nimpf, and W. J. Schneider. "Role of Leptin in Reproduction." *Current Opinion Lipidology* 15, no. 3 (June 2004): 315–19.

Baranowska, B., M. Radzikowska, E. Wasilewska-Dziubinska, A. Kaplinski, K. Roguski, and A. Plonowski. "Neuropeptide Y, Leptin, Galanin and Insulin in Women with Polycystic Ovary Syndrome." *Gynecological Endocrinology* 13, no. 5 (October 1999): 344–51.

Bayraktar, F., D. Dereli, A. G. Ozgen, and C. Yilmaz. "Plasma Homocysteine Levels in Polycystic Ovary Syndrome and Congenital Adrenal Hyperplasia." *Endocrinology Journal* 51, no. 6 (December 2004): 601–8.

Buccola, J. M., and E. E. Reynolds. "Polycystic Ovary Syndrome: A Review for Primary Providers." *Primary Care* 30, no. 4 (December 2003): 697–710.

Clark, A. M., B. Thornley, L. Tomlinson, C. Galletley, and R. J. Norman. "Weight Loss in Obese Infertile Women Results in Improvement in Reproductive Outcome for All Forms of Fertility Treatment." *Human Reproduction* 13, no. 6 (June 1998): 1502–5.

Fedorcsak, P., P. O. Dale, R. Storeng, G. Ertzeid, S. Bjercke, N. Oldereid, A. K. Omland, T. Abyholm, and T. Tanbo. "Impact of Overweight and Underweight on Assisted Reproduction Treatment." *Human Reproduction* 19, no. 11 (November 2004): 2523–28.

Goodarzi, M. O., S. Erickson, S. C. Port, R. I. Jennrich, and S. G. Korenman. "Beta-Cell Function: A Key Pathological Determinant in Polycystic Ovary Syndrome." *Journal of Clinical Endocrinology and Metabolism* 90, no. 1 (January 2005): 310–15.

Goumenou, A. G., I. M. Matalliotakis, G. E. Koumantakis, and D. K. Panidis. "The Role of Leptin in Fertility." *European Journal of Obstetrics and Gynecology and Reproductive Biology* 106, no. 2 (February 2003): 118–24.

Grodstein, F., M. B. Goldman, and D. W. Cramer. "Body Mass Index and Ovulatory Infertility." *Epidemiology* 5, no. 2 (March 1994): 247–50.

Grundy, S. "Inflammation, Metabolic Syndrome, and Diet Responsiveness." *Circulation* 108 (2003): 126.

Halis, G., and A. Arici. "Endometriosis and Inflammation in Infertility." *Annals of the New York Academy of Science* 1034 (December 2004): 300–315.

Hu, F. B. "Overweight and Obesity in Women: Health Risks and Consequences." *Journal of Women's Health* 12, no. 2 (March 2003): 163–72.

Kalro, B. N. "Impaired Fertility Caused by Endocrine Dysfunction in Women." *Endocrinology and Metabolism Clinics of North America* 32, no. 3 (September 2003): 573–92.

Kirchengast, S., and J. Huber. "Body Composition Characteristics and Fat Distribution Patterns in Young Infertile Women." *Fertility and Sterility* 81, no. 3 (March 2004): 539–44.

Lee, R. M., M. A. Brown, K. Ward, L. Nelson, D. W. Branch, and R. M. Silver. "Homocysteine Levels in Women with Antiphospholipid Syndrome and Normal Fertile Controls." *Journal of Reproductive Immunology* 63, no. 1 (August 2004): 23–30.

Lee, Y. H., and R. E. Pratley. "The Evolving Role of Inflammation in Obesity and the Metabolic Syndrome." *Current Diabetes Reports* 5, no. 1 (February 2005): 70–75.

Lopez-Garcia, E., M. B. Schulze, T. T. Fung, J. B. Meigs, N. Rifai, J. E. Manson, and F. B. Hu. "Major Dietary Patterns Are Related to Plasma Concentrations of Markers of Inflammation and Endothelial Dysfunction." *American Journal of Clinical Nutrition* 80, no. 4 (October 2004): 1029–35.

Marshall, K. "Polycystic Ovary Syndrome: Clinical Considerations." *Alternative Medicine Review* 6, no. 3 (June 2001): 272–92.

Messinis, I. E., and S. D. Milingos. "Leptin in Human Reproduction." *Human Reproduction Update* 5, no. 1 (January–February 1999): 52–63.

Moran, L., and R. J. Norman. "Understanding and Managing Disturbances in Insulin Metabolism and Body Weight in Women with

Polycystic Ovary Syndrome." *Best Practice and Research. Clinical Obstetrics and Gynaecology* 18, no. 5 (October 2004): 719–36.

Moran, L. J., M. Noakes, P. M. Clifton, G. A. Wittert, L. Tomlinson, C. Galletly, N. D. Luscombe, and R. J. Norman. "Ghrelin and Measures of Satiety Are Altered in Polycystic Ovary Syndrome but Not Differentially Affected by Diet Composition." *Journal of Clinical Endocrinology and Metabolism* 89, no. 7 (July 2004): 3337–44.

Norman, R. J., and A. M. Clark. "Obesity and Reproductive Disorders: A Review." *Reproduction, Fertility, and Development* 10, no. 1 (1998): 55–63.

Norman, R. J., M. Noakes, R. Wu, M. J. Davies, L. Moran, and J. X. Wang. "Improving Reproductive Performance in Overweight/Obese Women with Effective Weight Management." *Human Reproduction Update* 10, no. 3 (May–June 2004): 267–80.

Orio, F., Jr., P. Lucidi, S. Palomba, L. Tauchmanova, T. Cascella, T. Russo, F. Zullo, A. Colao, G. Lombardi, and P. De Feo. "Circulating Ghrelin Concentrations in the Polycystic Ovary Syndrome." *Journal of Clinical Endocrinology and Metabolism* 88, no. 2 (February 2003): 942–45.

Pasquali, R., F. Casimirri, S. Venturoli, M. Antonio, L. Morselli, S. Reho, A. Pezzoli, and R. Paradisi. "Body Fat Distribution Has Weight-Independent Effects on Clinical, Hormonal, and Metabolic Features of Women with Polycystic Ovary Syndrome." *Metabolism* 43, no. 6 (June 1994): 706–13.

Pasquali, R., C. Pelusi, S. Genghini, M. Cacciari, and A. Gambineri. "Obesity and Reproductive Disorders in Women." *Human Reproduction Update* 9, no. 4 (July–August 2003): 359–72.

Pischon, T., C. J. Girman, N. Rifai, G. S. Hotamisligil, and E. B. Rimm. "Association Between Dietary Factors and Plasma Adiponectin Concentrations in Men." *American Journal of Clinical Nutrition* 81, no. 4 (April 2005): 780–86.

Roberts, J. M., and P. Speer. "Antioxidant Therapy to Prevent Preeclampsia." *Seminar in Nephrology* 24, no. 6 (November 2004): 557–64.

Schroder, A. K., S. Tauchert, O. Ortmann, K. Diedrich, and J. M. Weiss. "Insulin Resistance in Patients with Polycystic Ovary Syndrome." *Annals of Medicine* 36, no. 6 (2004): 426–39.

Spranger, J., M. Mohlig, U. Wegewitz, M. Ristow, A. F. Pfeiffer, T. Schillt, H. W. Schlosser, G. Brabant, and C. Schofl. "Adiponectin Is Independently Associated with Insulin Sensitivity in Women with Polycystic Ovary Syndrome." *Obstetrical and Gynecological Survey* 60, no. 4 (April 2005): 237–39.

Wang, J. X., M. J. Davies, and R. J. Norman. "Obesity Increases the Risk of Spontaneous Abortion During Infertility Treatment." *Obesity Research* 10, no. 6 (June 2002): 551–54.

Yilmaz, M., N. Bukan, R. Ersoy, A. Karakoc, I. Yetkin, G. Ayvaz, N. Cakir, and M. Arslan. "Glucose Intolerance, Insulin Resistance and Cardiovascular Risk Factors in First Degree Relatives of Women with Polycystic Ovary Syndrome." *Human Reproduction* 2005 May 12; [Epub ahead of print].

Chapter 3: Fats, Carbs, and Your Fertility

Abayasekara, D. R., and D. C. Wathes. "Effects of Altering Dietary Fatty Acid Composition on Prostaglandin Synthesis and Fertility." *Prostaglandins, Leukotrienes, and Essential Fatty Acids* 61, no. 5 (November 1999): 275–87.

Ajani, U. A., E. S. Ford, and A. H. Mokdad. "Dietary Fiber and C-Reactive Protein: Findings from National Health and Nutrition Examination Survey Data." *Journal of Nutrition* 134, no. 5 (May 2004): 1181–85.

Anderson, J. W., N. J. Gustafson, C. A. Bryant, and J. Tietyen-Clark. "Dietary Fiber and Diabetes: A Comprehensive Review and Practical Application." *Journal of the American Dietetic Association* 87 (1987): 1189–97.

Anderson, N. K., K. A. Beerman, M. A. McGuire, N. Dasgupta, J. M. Griinari, J. Williams, and M. K. McGuire. "Dietary Fat Type Influences Total Milk Fat Content in Lean Women." *Journal of Nutrition* 135, no. 3 (March 2005): 416–21.

Baer, D. J., J. T. Judd, B. A. Clevidence, and R. P. Tracy. "Dietary Fatty Acids Affect Plasma Markers of Inflammation in Healthy Men Fed Controlled Diets: A Randomized Crossover Study." *American Journal of Clinical Nutrition* 79, no. 6 (June 2004): 969–73.

Bantle, J. "Clinical Aspects of Sucrose and Fructose Metabolism." *Diabetes Care* 12 (1984): 56–61.

Berry, E. M. "Dietary Fatty Acids in the Management of Diabetes Mellitus." *American Journal of Clinical Nutrition* 66, 4 supplement (October 1997): 991S–997S.

Brand, J. C., P. L. Nicholson, A. W. Thorburn, and A. S. Truswell. "Food Processing and the Glycemic Index." *American Journal of Clinical Nutrition* 42, no. 6 (1985): 1192–96.

Covens, A. L., P. Christopher, and R. F. Casper. "The Effect of Dietary Supplementation with Fish Oil Fatty Acids on Surgically Induced Endometriosis in the Rabbit." *Fertility and Sterility* 49, no. 4 (April 1988): 698–703.

Decsi, T., and B. Koletzko. "N-3 Fatty Acids and Pregnancy Outcomes." *Current Opinion in Clinical Nutrition and Metabolic Care* 8, no. 2 (March 2005): 161–66.

Edmond, J. "Essential Polyunsaturated Fatty Acids and the Barrier to the Brain: The Components of a Model for Transport." *Journal of Molecular Neuroscience* 16, nos. 2–3 (April–June 2001): 181–93, discussion 215–21.

Facchinetti, F., M. Fazzio, and P. Venturini. "Polyunsaturated Fatty Acids and Risk of Preterm Delivery." *European Review for Medical and Pharmacological Sciences* 9, no. 1 (January–February 2005): 41–48.

Ford, E. S., A. H. Mokdad, and S. Liu. "Healthy Eating Index and C-Reactive Protein Concentration: Findings from the National Health and Nutrition Examination Survey III, 1988-1994." *European Journal of Clinical Nutrition* 59, no. 2 (February 2005): 278–83.

Fung, T. T., F. B. Hu, M. A. Pereira, et al. "Whole-Grain Intake and the Risk of Type 2 Diabetes: A Prospective Study in Men." *American Journal of Clinical Nutrition* 76 (2002): 535–40.

Gazvani, M. R., L. Smith, P. Haggarty, P. A. Fowler, and A. Templeton. "High Omega-3: Omega-6 Fatty Acid Ratios in Culture Medium Reduce Endometrial-Cell Survival in Combined Endometrial Gland and Stromal Cell Cultures from Women with and Without Endometriosis." *Fertility and Sterility* 76, no. 4 (October 2001): 717–22.

Gillen, L. J., and L. C. Tapsell. "Advice That Includes Food Sources of Unsaturated Fat Supports Future Risk Management of Gestational Diabetes Mellitus." *Journal of the American Dietetic Association* 104, no. 12 (December 2004): 1863–67.

Hallfrisch, J., and K. M. Behall. "Mechanisms of the Effects of Grains on Insulin and Glucose Responses." *Journal of the American College of Nutrition* 19 (3 supplement) (2000): 320S–325S.

"Health Implications of Dietary Fiber." Position of ADA *Journal of the American Dietetic Association* 97 (1997): 1157–59.

Helland, I. B., L. Smith, K. Saarem, O. D. Saugstad, and C. A. Drevon. "Maternal Supplementation with Very-Long-Chain n-3 Fatty Acids During Pregnancy and Lactation Augments Children's IQ at 4 Years of Age." *Pediatrics* 111, no. 1 (January 2003): e39–44.

Ibrahim, A., S. Natrajan, and R. Ghafoorunissa. "Dietary Trans-Fatty Acids Alter Adipocyte Plasma Membrane Fatty Acid Composition and Insulin Sensitivity in Rats." *Metabolism* 54, no. 2 (February 2005): 240–46.

Jalili, T., R. E. C. Wildman, and D. M. Medeiros. "Nutraceutical Roles of Dietary Fiber." *Journal of Nutraceuticals, Functional, and Medical Foods* 2, no. 4 (2000): 19–34.

Jenkins, D. J., C. W. Kendall, L. S. Augustin, et al. "Glycemic Index: Overview of Implications in Health and Disease." *American Journal of Clinical Nutrition* 76 (2002): 266S–273S.

Kasim-Karakas, S. E., R. U. Almario, L. Gregory, R. Wong, H. Todd, and B. L. Lasley. "Metabolic and Endocrine Effects of a Polyunsaturated Fatty Acid–Rich Diet in Polycystic Ovary Syndrome." *Journal of Clinical Endocrinology and Metabolism* 89, no. 2 (February 2004): 615–20.

Khor, G. L. "Dietary Fat Quality: A Nutritional Epidemiologist's View." *Asia Pacific Journal of Clinical Nutrition* 13, supplement (August 2004): S22.

King, D. E., B. M. Egan, and M. E. Geesey. "Relation of Dietary Fat and Fiber to Elevation of C-Reactive Protein." *American Journal of Cardiology* 92, no. 11 (December 1, 2003): 1335–39.

Korotkova, M., B. G. Gabrielsson, A. Holmang, B. M. Larsson, L. A. Hanson, and B. Strandvik. "Gender-Related Long-Term Effects in Adult Rats by Perinatal Dietary Ratio of n-6/n-3 Fatty Acids." *American Journal of Physiology—Regulatory, Integrative, and Comparative Physiology* 288, no. 3 (March 2005): R575–79.

Lichtenstein, A. H., A. T. Erkkila, B. Lamarche, U. S. Schwab, S. M. Jalbert, and L. M. Ausman. "Influence of Hydrogenated Fat and Butter on CVD Risk Factors: Remnant-Like Particles, Glucose and Insulin, Blood Pressure and C-Reactive Protein." *Atherosclerosis* 171, no. 1 (November 2003): 97–107.

Liese, A. D., M. Schulz, C. G. Moore, and E. J. Mayer-Davis. "Dietary Patterns, Insulin Sensitivity and Adiposity in the Multi-Ethnic Insulin Resistance Atherosclerosis Study Population." *British Journal of Nutrition* 92, no. 6 (December 2004): 973–84.

Liu, S., W. C. Willett, J. E. Manson, F. B. Hu, B. Rosner, and G. Colditz. "Relation Between Changes in Intakes of Dietary Fiber and Grain Products and Changes in Weight and Development of Obesity Among Middle-Aged Women." *American Journal of Clinical Nutrition* 78, no. 5 (November 2003): 920–27.

Liu, S., W. C. Willett, P. M. Ridker, J. E. Manson, J. E. Buring, and M. J. Stampfer. "Relation Between a Diet with a High Glycemic Load and Plasma Concentrations of High-Sensitivity C-Reactive Protein in Middle-Aged Women." *American Journal of Clinical Nutrition* 75, no. 3 (March 2002): 492–98.

Liu, S., W. C. Willett, M. J. Stampfer, et al. "A Prospective Study of Dietary Glycemic Load, Carbohydrate Intake, and Risk of Coronary Heart Disease in U.S. Women." *American Journal of Clinical Nutrition* 71 (2000): 1455–61.

Liu, S. "Insulin Resistance, Hyperglycemia and Risk of Major Chronic Diseases—a Dietary Perspective." *Proceedings of the Nutrition Society of Australia* 22 (1998): 140–50.

Liu, S. "Intake of Refined Carbohydrates and Whole Grain Foods in Relation to Risk of Type 2 Diabetes Mellitus and Coronary Heart Disease." *Journal of the American College of Nutrition* 21, no. 4 (2002): 298–306.

Loosemore, E. D., M. P. Judge, and C. J. Lammi-Keefe. "Dietary Intake of Essential and Long-Chain Polyunsaturated Fatty Acids in Pregnancy." *Lipids* 39, no. 5 (May 2004): 421–24.

Lopez-Garcia, E., M. B. Schulze, J. B. Meigs, J. E. Manson, N. Rifai, M. J. Stampfer, W. C. Willett, and F. B. Hu. "Consumption of Trans Fatty Acids Is Related to Plasma Biomarkers of Inflammation and Endothelial Dysfunction." *Journal of Nutrition* 135, no. 3 (March 2005): 562–66.

Louheranta, A. M., E. S. Sarkkinen, H. M. Vidgren, U. S. Schwab, and M. I. Uusitupa. "Association of the Fatty Acid Profile of Serum Lipids with Glucose and Insulin Metabolism During 2 Fat-Modified Diets in Subjects with Impaired Glucose Tolerance." *American Journal of Clinical Nutrition* 76, no. 2 (August 2002): 331–37.

Ludwig, D. S. "Diet and Development of Insulin Resistance Syndrome." *Asia Pacific Journal of Clinical Nutrition* 12 supplement (2003): S4.

Ludwig, D. "Dietary Glycemic Index and Obesity." *Journal of Nutrition* 130 (2000): 280S–283S.

Manco, M., M. Calvani, and G. Mingrone. "Effects of Dietary Fatty Acids on Insulin Sensitivity and Secretion." *Diabetes, Obesity, and Metabolism* 6, no. 6 (November 2004): 402–13.

Marlett, J. A., M. I. McBurney, J. L. Slavin, and the American Dietetic Association. "Position of the American Dietetic Association: Health

Implications of Dietary Fiber." *Journal of the American Dietetic Association* 102, no. 7 (July 2002): 993–1000.

Marlett, J. A. "Content and Composition of Dietary Fiber in 117 Frequently Consumed Foods." *Journal of American Dietetic Association* 92 (1992): 175–86.

Matorras, R., J. I. Ruiz, R. Mendoza, N. Ruiz, P. Sanjurjo, and F. J. Rodriguez-Escudero. "Fatty Acid Composition of Fertilization-Failed Human Oocytes." *Human Reproduction* 13, no. 8 (August 1998): 2227–30.

McKeown, N. M., J. B. Meigs, S. Liu, E. Saltzman, P. W. Wilson, and P. F. Jacques. "Carbohydrate Nutrition, Insulin Resistance, and the Prevalence of the Metabolic Syndrome in the Framingham Offspring Cohort." *Diabetes Care* 27 (2004): 538–46.

McKeown, N. M., J. B. Meigs, S. Liu, P. W. Wilson, and P. F. Jacques. "Whole-Grain Intake Is Favorably Associated with Metabolic Risk Factors for Type 2 Diabetes and Cardiovascular Disease in the Framingham Offspring Study." *American Journal of Clinical Nutrition* 76, no. 2 (August 2002): 390–98.

Mozaffarian, D., T. Pischon, S. E. Hankinson, N. Rifai, K. Joshipura, W. C. Willett, and E. B. Rimm. "Dietary Intake of Trans Fatty Acids and Systemic Inflammation in Women." *American Journal of Clinical Nutrition* 79, no. 4 (April 2004): 606–12.

Mozaffarian, D., E. B. Rimm, I. B. King, R. L. Lawler, G. B. McDonald, and W. C. Levy. "Trans Fatty Acids and Systemic Inflammation in Heart Failure." *American Journal of Clinical Nutrition* 80, no. 6 (December 2004): 1521–25.

U.S. Food and Drug Administration, Center for Food Safety and Applied Nutrition. Questions and Answers on Trans Fat Proposed Rule. November 1999.

Rustan, A. C., M. S. Nenseter, and C. A. Drevon. "Omega-3 and Omega-6 Fatty Acids in the Insulin Resistance Syndrome. Lipid and Lipoprotein Metabolism and Atherosclerosis." *Annals of the New York Academy of Sciences* 827, no. 1 (1997): 310–26.

Saldeen, P., and T. Saldeen. "Women and Omega-3 Fatty Acids." *Obstetrical and Gynecological Survey* 59, no. 10 (October 2004): 722–30, quiz 745–46.

Schulze, M. B., S. Liu, E. B. Rimm, J. E. Manson, W. C. Willett, and F. B. Hu. "Glycemic Index, Glycemic Load, and Dietary Fiber Intake and Incidence of Type 2 Diabetes in Younger and Middle-Aged Women." *American Journal of Clinical Nutrition* 80 (2004): 348–56.

Simopoulos, A. P. "Essential Fatty Acids in Health and Chronic Disease." *American Journal of Clinical Nutrition* 70, 3 supplement (September 1999): 560S–569S.

Sir-Petermann, T., B. Angel, M. Maliqueo, J. L. Santos, M. V. Riesco, H. Toloza, and F. Perez-Bravo. "Insulin Secretion in Women Who Have Polycystic Ovary Syndrome and Carry the Gly972Arg Variant of Insulin Receptor Substrate-1 in Response to a High-Glycemic or Low-Glycemic Carbohydrate Load." *Nutrition* 20, no. 10 (October 2004): 905–10.

Song, Y., J. E. Manson, J. E. Buring, and S. Liu. "A Prospective Study of Red Meat Consumption and Type 2 Diabetes in Middle-Aged and Elderly Women: The Women's Health Study." *Diabetes Care* 27, no. 9 (September 2004): 2108–15.

Stark, A. H., and Z. Madar. "Olive Oil as a Functional Food: Epidemiology and Nutritional Approaches." *Nutrition Review* 60, no. 6 (June 2002): 170–76.

Thorne, M. J., L. U. Thompson, and D. J. Jenkins. "Factors Affecting Starch Digestibility and the Glycemic Response with Special Reference to Legumes." *American Journal of Clinical Nutrition* 38 (1983): 481–88.

van Dam, R. M., W. C. Willett, E. B. Rimm, M. J. Stampfer, and F. B. Hu. "Dietary Fat and Meat Intake in Relation to Risk of Type 2 Diabetes in Men." *Diabetes Care* 25, no. 3 (March 2002): 417–24.

Veldman, F. J., C. H. Nair, H. H. Vorster, et al. "Dietary Pectin Influences Fibrin Network Structure in Hypercholesterolaemic Subjects." *Thrombosis Research* 86 (1997): 183–96.

Whalley, L. J., H. C. Fox, K. W. Wahle, J. M. Starr, and I. J. Deary. "Cognitive Aging, Childhood Intelligence, and the Use of Food Supplements: Possible Involvement of n-3 Fatty Acids." *American Journal of Clinical Nutrition* 80, no. 6 (December 2004): 1650–57.

Wolever, T., and C. Bolognesi. "Prediction of Glucose and Insulin Responses of Normal Subjects After Consuming Mixed Meals Varying in Energy, Protein, Fat, Carbohydrate and Glycemic Index." *Nutrition* 126 (1992): 2807–12.

Wolever, T., L. Katzman-Relle, A. L. Jenkins, et al. "Glycemic Index of 102 Complex Carbohydrate Foods in Patients with Diabetes." *Nutritional Research* 14 (1994): 651–69.

Wolever, T. M., D. J. Jenkins, A. L. Jenkins, and R. G. Josse. "The Glycemic Index: Methodology and Clinical Implications." *American Journal of Clinical Nutrition* 54, no. 5 (1991): 846–54.

Chapter 4: Antioxidants, Phytonutrients, and Other Fertility-Boosting Nutrients

Avena, R., A. Arora, B. J. Carmody, K. Cosby, and A. N. Sidawy. "Thiamine (Vitamin B$_1$) Protects Against Glucose- and Insulin-Mediated Proliferation of Human Infragenicular Arterial Smooth Muscle Cells." *Annals of Vascular Surgery* 14, no. 1 (January 2000): 37–43.

Babu, P. S., and K. Srinivasan. "Influence of Dietary Curcumin and Cholesterol on the Progression of Experimentally Induced Diabetes in Albino Rat." *Molecular and Cellular Biochemistry* 152, no. 1 (November 8, 1995): 13–21.

Baltaci, A. K., R. Mogulkoc, and I. Halifeoglu. "Effects of Zinc Deficiency and Supplementation on Plasma Leptin Levels in Rats." *Biological Trace Element Research* 104, no. 1 (April 2005): 41–46.

Barbagallo, M., L. J. Dominguez, M. R. Tagliamonte, L. M. Resnick, and G. Paolisso. "Effects of Vitamin E and Glutathione on Glucose Metabolism: Role of Magnesium." *Hypertension* 34, no. 4 pt. 2 (October 1999): 1002–6.

Beckett, G. J., and J. R. Arthur. "Selenium and Endocrine Systems." *Journal of Endocrinology* 184, no. 3 (March 2005): 455–65.

Bhathena, S. J., and M. T. Velasquez. "Beneficial Role of Dietary Phytoestrogens in Obesity and Diabetes." *American Journal of Clinical Nutrition* 76, no. 6 (December 2002): 1191–1201.

Bo, S., A. Lezo, G. Menato, M. L. Gallo, C. Bardelli, A. Signorile, C. Berutti, M. Massobrio, and G. F. Pagano. "Gestational Hyperglycemia, Zinc, Selenium, and Antioxidant Vitamins." *Nutrition* 21, no. 2 (February 2005): 186–91.

Bordia, A., S. K. Verma, and K. C. Srivastava. "Effect of Garlic (*Allium sativum*) on Blood Lipids, Blood Sugar, Fibrinogen and Fibrinolytic Activity in Patients with Coronary Artery Disease." *Prostaglandins, Leukotrienes, and Essential Fatty Acids* 58, no. 4 (April 1998): 257–63.

Centers for Disease Control and Prevention. *Centers for Disease Control and Prevention: Diabetes Surveillance Report.* Atlanta: Department of Health and Human Services, 1999.

Cho, S. Y., S. J. Park, M. J. Kwon, T. S. Jeong, S. H. Bok, W. Y. Choi, W. I. Jeong, S. Y. Ryu, S. H. Do, C. S. Lee, J. C. Song, and K. S. Jeong. "Quercetin Suppresses Proinflammatory Cytokines Production Through MAP Kinases and NF-kappaB Pathway in Lipopolysaccharide-Stimulated Macrophage." *Molecular and Cellular Biochemistry* 243, nos. 1–2 (January 2003): 153–60.

Cohen-Boulakia, F., P. E. Valensi, H. Boulahdour, R. Lestrade, J. F. Dufour-Lamartinie, C. Hort-Legrand, and A Behar. "In Vivo Sequential Study of Skeletal Muscle Capillary Permeability in Diabetic Rats: Effect of Anthocyanosides." *Metabolism* 49, no. 7 (July 2000): 880–85.

Coskun, O., M. Kanter, A. Korkmaz, and S. Oter. "Quercetin, a Flavonoid Antioxidant, Prevents and Protects Streptozotocin-Induced Oxidative Stress and Beta-Cell Damage in Rat Pancreas." *Pharmacological Research* 51, no. 2 (February 2005): 117–23.

Cowell, R. C., and J. W. Russell. "Nirosaative Injury and Antioxidant Therapy in the Management of Diabetic Neuropathy." *Journal of Investigative Medicine* 52 (2004): 33–44.

Davi, G., G. Ciabattoni, A. Consoli, et al. "In Vivo Formation of 8-iso-Prostaglandin F2a and Platelet Activation in Diabetes Mellitus. Effects of Improved Metabolic Control and Vitamin E Supplementation." *Circulation* 99 (1999): 224–29.

Debier, C., and Y. Larondelle. "Vitamins A and E: Metabolism, Roles and Transfer to Offspring." *British Journal of Nutrition* 93, no. 2 (February 2005): 153–74.

Dickinson, P. J., A. L. Carrington, G. S. Frost, and A. J. Boutlon. "Neurovascular Disease, Antioxidants and Glycation in Diabetes." *Diabetes/Metabolism Research and Reviews* 18, no. 4 (July–August 2002): 260–72.

Dixon, R. A. "Phytoestrogens." *Annual Review of Plant Biology* 55 (2004): 225–61.

Elkayam, A., D. Mirelman, E. Peleg, M. Wilchek, T. Miron, A. Rabinkov, M. Oron-Herman, and T. Rosenthal. "The Effects of Allicin on Weight in Fructose-Induced Hyperinsulinemic, Hyperlipidemic, Hypertensive Rats." *American Journal of Hypertension* 16, no. 12 (December 2003): 1053–56.

Exner, M., M. Hermann, R. Hofbauer, S. Kapiotis, P. Quehenberger, W. Speiser, I. Held, and B. M. Gmeiner. "Genistein Prevents the Glucose Autoxidation Mediated Atherogenic Modification of Low Density Lipoprotein." *Free Radical Research* 34, no. 1 (January 2001): 101–12.

Freund, H., I. J. Benjamin, G. L. Burke, et al. "Chromium Deficiency During Total Parenteral Nutrition." *JAMA* 241, no. 5 (1979): 496–98.

Fugh-Berman, A., and F. Kronenberg. "Complementary and Alternative Medicine (CAM) in Reproductive-Age Women: A Review of Randomized Controlled Trials." *Reproductive Toxicology* 17, no. 2 (March–April 2003): 137–52.

Haskins, K., J. Kench, K. Powers, B. Bradley, S. Pugazhenthi, and J. Reusch. "Role for Oxidative Stress in the Regeneration of Islet Beta Cells?" *Journal of Investigative Medicine* 52 (2004): 45–49.

Heber, D. "Vegetables, Fruits and Phytoestrogens in the Prevention of Diseases." *Journal of Postgraduate Medicine* 50, no. 2 (April–June 2004): 145–49.

Heber, D., and S. Bowerman. "Applying Science to Changing Dietary Patterns." *Journal of Nutrition* 131 (November 2001): 3078S–3081S.

Herzog, A., U. Siler, V. Spitzer, N. Seifert, A. Denelavas, P. B. Hunziker, W. Hunziker, R. Goralczyk, and K. Wertz. "Lycopene Reduced Gene Expression of Steroid Targets and Inflammatory Markers in Normal Rat Prostate." *The FASEB Journal* 19, no. 2 (February 2005): 272–74.

Ho, E., and T. M. Bray. "Antioxidants, NFkappaB Activation, and Diabetogenesis." *Proceedings of the Society for Experimental Biology and Medicine* 222 (1999): 205–13.

Huang, C. N., J. S. Horng, and M. C. Yin. "Antioxidative and Antiglycative Effects of Six Organosulfur Compounds in Low-Density Lipoprotein and Plasma." *Journal of Agricultural and Food Chemistry* 52, no. 11 (June 2004): 3674–78.

Jung, W. J., and M. K. Sung. "Effects of Major Dietary Antioxidants on Inflammatory Markers of RAW 264.7 Macrophages." *Biofactors* 21, nos. 1–4 (2004): 113–17.

Kaneto, H., Y. Kajimoto, Y. Fujitani, et al. "Oxidative Stress Induces p21 Expression in Pancreatic Islet Cells: Possible Implication in Beta-Cell Dysfunction." *Diabetologia* 42 (1999): 1093–97.

Khamaisi, M., O. Kavel, M. Rosenstock, M. Porat, M. Yuli, N. Kaiser, and A. Rudich. "Effect of Inhibition of Glutathione Synthesis on Insulin Action: In Vivo and In Vitro Studies Using Buthioninesulfoximine." *Biochemistry Journal* 349, pt. 2 (July 15, 2000): 579–86.

Kilicdag, E. B., T. Bagis, E. Tarim, E. Aslan, S. Erkanli, E. Simsek, B. Haydardedeoglu, and E. Kuscu. "Administration of B-Group Vitamins Reduces Circulating Homocysteine in Polycystic Ovarian Syn-

drome Patients Treated with Metformin: A Randomized Trial."
Human Reproduction 20, no. 6 (June 2005): 1521–28.

Knekt, P., J. Kumpulainen, R. Jarvinen, H. Rissanen, M. Heliovaara,
A. Reunanen, T. Hakulinen, and A. Aromaa. "Flavonoid Intake and
Risk of Chronic Diseases." *American Journal of Clinical Nutrition*
76, no. 3 (September 2002): 560–68.

Lampeter, E. F., A. Klinghammer, W. A. Scherbaum, et al. "The
Deutsche Nicotinamide Intervention Study: An Attempt to Prevent
Type 1 Diabetes." *Diabetes* 47 (1998): 980–84.

Liu, S. "Insulin Resistance, Hyperglycemia and Risk of Major Chronic
Diseases—a Dietary Perspective." *Proceedings of the Nutrition Society of Australia* 22 (1998): 140–50.

Liu, R. H. "Health Benefits of Fruits and Vegetables Are from Addi-
tive and Synergistic Combination of Phytochemicals." *American
Journal of Clinical Nutrition* 78 (2003): 517S–520S.

Luberda, Z. "The Role of Glutathione in Mammalian Gametes."
Reproductive Biology 5, no. 1 (March 2005): 5–17.

McDermott, J. H. "Antioxidant Nutrients: Current Dietary Recommendations and Research Update. *Journal of the American Pharmacological Association* 40, no. 6 (November–December 2000): 785–99.

Mezei, O., W. J. Banz, R. W. Steger, et al. "Soy Isoflavones Exert
Antidiabetic and Hypolipidemic Effects Through PPAR Pathways
in Obese Zucker Rats and Murine RAW 264.7 Cells." *Journal of
Nutrition* 133, no. 5 (May 2003): 1238–43.

Michnovicz, J. J., and H. L. Bradlow. "Altered Estrogen Metabolism
and Excretion in Humans Following Consumption of Indole
Carbinol." *Nutrition and Cancer* 16 (1991): 59–66.

Montonen, J., P. Knekt, R. Jarvinen, and A. Reunanen. "Dietary
Antioxidant Intake and Risk of Type 2 Diabetes." *Diabetes Care* 27,
no. 2 (February 2004): 362–66.

NCI, 5-A-Day Website, Glossary of Phytochemicals. 5aday.gov.

Ou, C. C., S. M. Tsao, M. C. Lin, and M. C. Yin. "Protective Action
on Human LDL Against Oxidation and Glycation by Four

Organosulfur Compounds Derived from Garlic." *Lipids* 38, no. 3 (March 2003): 219–24.

Paolisso, G., and M. Barbagallo. "Hypertension, Diabetes Mellitus, and Insulin Resistance: The Role of Intracellular Magnesium." *Journal of Hypertension* 10, no. 3 (1997): 346–55.

Pasquali, R., and A. Gambineri. "Role of Changes in Dietary Habits in Polycystic Ovary Syndrome." *Reproductive Biomedicine Online* 8, no. 4 (April 2004): 431–39.

Poston, L., M. Raijmakers, and F. Kelly. "Vitamin E in Preeclampsia." *Annals of the New York Academy of Sciences* 1031 (December 2004): 242–48.

Robertson, P. "Chronic Oxidative Stress as a Mechanism for Glucose Toxicity in Pancreatic Islet Beta Cells in Diabetes." *Journal of Biological Chemistry* 279, no. 41 (2004): 42351–54.

Romero-Navarro, G., G. Cabrera-Valladares, M. S. German, et al. "Biotin Regulation of Pancreatic Glucokinase and Insulin in Primary Cultured Rat Islets and in Biotin-Deficient Rats." *Endocrinology* 140 (1999): 4595–600.

Sekiya, K., A. Ohtani, and S. Kusano. "Enhancement of Insulin Sensitivity in Adipocytes by Ginger." *Biofactors* 22, nos. 1–4 (2004): 153–56.

Shi, J., K. Arunasalam, D. Yeung, Y. Kakuda, G. Mittal, and Y. Jiang. "Saponins from Edible Legumes: Chemistry, Processing, and Health Benefits." *Journal of Medicinal Food* 7, no. 1 (Spring 2004): 67–78.

Sidhu, G. S., H. Mani, J. P. Gaddipati, A. K. Singh, P. Seth, K. K. Banaudha, G. K. Patnaik, and R. K. Maheshwari. "Curcumin Enhances Wound Healing in Streptozotocin Induced Diabetic Rats and Genetically Diabetic Mice." *Wound Repair and Regeneration* 7, no. 5 (September–October 1999): 362–74.

Thompson, L. U., J. H. Yoon, D. J. Jenkins, T. M. Wolever, and A. L. Jenkins. "Relationship Between Polyphenol Intake and Blood Glucose Response of Normal and Diabetic Individuals." *American Journal of Clinical Nutrition* 38 (1984): 745–51.

Tijburg, L. B. M., T. Mattern, J. D. Folts, U. M. Weisgerber, and M. B. Katan. "Tea Flavonoids and Cardiovascular Diseases: A Review." *Critical Reviews in Food Science and Nutrition* 37 (1997): 771–85.

Ting, H. H., F. K. Timimi, K. S. Boles, S. J. Creager, P. Ganz, and M. A. Creager. "Vitamin C Improves Endothelium-Dependent Vasodilation in Patients with Non-Insulin-Dependent Diabetes Mellitus." *Journal of Clinical Investigation* 97 (1996): 22–28.

Tsuda, T., F. Horio, K. Uchida, H. Aoki, and T. Osawa. "Dietary Cyanidin 3-O-Beta-D-Glucoside-Rich Purple Corn Color Prevents Obesity and Ameliorates Hyperglycemia in Mice." *Journal of Nutrition* 133, no. 7 (July 2003): 2125–30.

Tsuda, T., Y. Ueno, H. Aoki, T. Koda, F. Horio, N. Takahashi, T. Kawada, and T. Osawa. "Anthocyanin Enhances Adipocytokine Secretion and Adipocyte-Specific Gene Expression in Isolated Rat Adipocytes." *Biochemical and Biophysical Research Communications* 316, no. 1 (March 26, 2004): 149–57.

United States Department of Agriculture, Agricultural Research Service (1998). "Food and Nutrient Intakes by Individuals in the United States, by Sex and Age, 1994–1996." Nationwide Food Surveys Report No. 96-2, 1998 USDA Washington, DC.

van Herpen-Broekmans, W. M., I. A. Klopping-Ketelaars, M. L. Bots, C. Kluft, H. Princen, H. F. Hendriks, L. B. Tijburg, G. van Poppel, and A. F. Kardinaal. "Serum Carotenoids and Vitamins in Relation to Markers of Endothelial Function and Inflammation." *European Journal of Epidemiology* 19, no. 10 (2004): 915–21.

Vaskonen, T. "Dietary Minerals and Modification of Cardiovascular Risk Factors." *Journal of Nutritional Biochemistry* 14, no. 9 (September 2003): 492–506.

Wahlberg, G., L. A. Carlson, J. Wasserman, et al. "Protective Effect of Nicotinamide Against Nephropathy in Diabetic Rats." *Diabetes Research* 2 (1985): 307.

Yeh, Y. Y., and L. Liu. "Cholesterol-Lowering Effect of Garlic Extracts and Organosulfur Compounds: Human and Animal Studies." *Journal of Nutrition* 131, no. 3s (March 2001): 989S–993S.

Zhang, H., K. Osada, H. Sone, et al. "Biotin Administration Improves the Impaired Glucose Tolerance of Streptozotocin-Induced Diabetic Wistar Rats." *Journal of Nutritional Science and Vitaminology* 43 (1997): 2271–280.

Chapter 5: For the Boys: Increasing Vitality Through Diet

Chen, Q., V. Ng, J. Mei, S. E. Chia. "Comparison of Seminal Vitamin B_{12}, Folate, Reactive Oxygen Species and Various Sperm Parameters Between Fertile and Infertile Males." *Wei Sheng Yan Jiu* 30, no. 2 (2001): 80–82.

Comhaire, F. H., and A. Mahmoud. "The Role of Food Supplements in the Treatment of the Infertile Man." *Reproductive Biomedicine Online* 7, no. 4 (October–November 2003): 385–91.

Eskenazi, B., S. A. Kidd, A. R. Marks, E. Sloter, G. Block, and A. J. Wyrobek. "Antioxidant Intake Is Associated with Semen Quality in Healthy Men." *Human Reproduction* 20, no. 4 (April 2005): 1006–12.

Eskiocak, S., A. S. Gozen, S. B. Yapar, F. Tavas, A. S. Kilic, and M. Eskiocak. "Glutathione and Free Sulphydryl Content of Seminal Plasma in Healthy Medical Students During and After Exam Stress." *Human Reproduction* 2005 May 12; [Epub ahead of print].

Foresta, C., L. Flohe, A. Garolla, A. Roveri, F. Ursini, and M. Maiorino. "Male Fertility Is Linked to the Selenoprotein Phospholipid Hydroperoxide Glutathione Peroxidase." *Biology of Reproduction* 67, no. 3 (September 2002): 967–71.

Greco, E., M. Iacobelli, L. Rienzi, F. Ubaldi, S. Ferrero, and J. Tesarik. "Reduction of the Incidence of Sperm DNA Fragmentation by Oral Antioxidant Treatment." *Journal of Andrology* 26, no. 3 (May–June 2005): 349–53.

Hawkes, W. C., and P. J. Turek. "Effects of Dietary Selenium on Sperm Motility in Healthy Men." *Journal of Andrology* 22, no. 5 (September–October 2001): 764–72.

Kaur, P., and M. P. Bansal. "Effect of Selenium-Induced Oxidative Stress on the Cell Kinetics in Testis and Reproductive Ability of Male Mice." *Nutrition* 21, no. 3 (March 2005): 351–57.

Koca, Y., O. L. Ozdal, M. Celik, S. Unal, and N. Balaban. "Antioxidant Activity of Seminal Plasma in Fertile and Infertile Men." *Archives of Andrology* 49, no. 5 (September–October 2003): 355–59.

Maiorino, M., and F. Ursini. "Oxidative Stress, Spermatogenesis and Fertility." *Journal of Biological Chemistry* 383, nos. 3–4 (March–April 2002): 591–97.

Ollero, M., E. Gil-Guzman, M. C. Lopez, R. K. Sharma, A. Agarwal, K. Larson, D. Evenson, A. J. Thomas Jr., and J. G. Alvarez. "Characterization of Subsets of Human Spermatozoa at Different Stages of Maturation: Implications in the Diagnosis and Treatment of Male Infertility." *Human Reproduction* 16, no. 9 (September 2001): 1912–21.

Sinclair, S. "Male Infertility: Nutritional and Environmental Considerations." *Alternative Medical Review* 5, no. 1 (February 2000): 28–38.

Su, D., S. V. Novoselov, Q. A. Sun, M. E. Moustafa, Y. Zhou, R. Oko, D. L. Hatfield, V. N. Gladyshev. "Mammalian Selenoprotein Thioredoxin/Glutathione Reductase: Roles in Disulfide Bond Formation and Sperm Maturation." *Journal of Biological Chemistry* 2005 May 18; [Epub ahead of print].

Wallock, L. M., T. Tamura, C. A. Mayr, K. E. Johnston, B. N. Ames, and R. A. Jacob. "Low Seminal Plasma Folate Concentrations Are Associated with Low Sperm Density and Count in Male Smokers and Nonsmokers." *Fertility and Sterility* 75, no. 2 (February 2001): 252–59.

Watanabe, T., K. Ohkawa, S. Kasai, S. Ebara, Y. Nakano, and Y. Watanabe. "The Effects of Dietary Vitamin B_{12} Deficiency on Sperm Maturation in Developing and Growing Male Rats." *Congenital Anomalies* (Kyoto) 43, no. 1 (March 2003): 57–64.

Wong, W. Y., H. M. Merkus, C. M. Thomas, R. Menkveld, G. A. Zielhuis, and R. P. Steegers-Theunissen. "Effects of Folic Acid and Zinc

Sulfate on Male Factor Subfertility: A Double-Blind, Randomized, Placebo-Controlled Trial." *Fertility and Sterility* 77, no. 3 (March 2002): 491–98.

Chapter 6: Foods to Be Fruitful

Adom, K. K. and R. H. Liu. "Antioxidant Activity of Grains." *Journal of Agricultural Food Chemistry* 50 (2002): 6182–87.

Adom, K. K., M. E. Sorrells, and R. H. Liu. "Phytochemicals and Antioxidant Activity of Wheat Varieties." *Journal of Agricultural Food Chemistry* 51 (2003): 7825–34.

Eberhardt, M. V., C. Y. Lee, and R. H. Liu "Antioxidant Activity of Fresh Apples." *Nature* 405 (2000): 903–4.

Gao, X., O. I. Bermudez, and K. L. Tucker. "Plasma C-Reactive Protein and Homocysteine Concentrations Are Related to Frequent Fruit and Vegetable Intake in Hispanic and Non-Hispanic White Elders." *Journal of Nutrition* 134, no. 4 (2004): 913–18.

Heber, D. "Vegetables, Fruits and Phytoestrogens in the Prevention of Diseases." *Journal of Postgraduate Medicine* 50 (2004): 145–49.

Jacobs, D., and L. Steffen. "Nutrients, Foods and Dietary Patterns as Exposures in Research: A Framework for Food Synergy." *American Journal of Clinical Nutrition* 78, 3 supplement (September 2003): 508S–513S.

Keiss, H. P., V. M. Dirsch, T. Hartung, T. Haffner, L. Trueman, J. Auger, R. Kahane, and A. M. Vollmar. "Garlic (*Allium sativum L.*) Modulates Cytokine Expression in Lipopolysaccharide-Activated Human Blood Thereby Inhibiting NF-KappaB Activity." *Journal of Nutrition* 133, no. 7 (July 2003): 2171–75.

Martinez-Dominguez, E., R. de la Puerta, and V. Ruiz-Gutierrez. "Protective Effects Upon Experimental Inflammation Models of a Polyphenol-Supplemented Virgin Olive Oil Diet." *Inflammation Research* 50, no. 2 (February 2001): 102–6.

Ommen, G. S., G. E. Goodman, M. D. Thomquist, J. Barnes, and M. R. Cullen. "Effects of a Combination of ß-Carotene and Vitamin A on Lung Cancer and Cardiovascular Disease." *New England Journal of Medicine* 334 (1996): 1150–55.

Salonen, J. T., K. Nyyssonen, R. Salonen, H. M. Lakka, J. Kaikkonen, E. Porkkala-Sarataho, S. Voutilainen, T. A. Lakka, T. Rissanen, et al. "Antioxidant Supplementation in Artherosclerosis Prevention (ASAP) Study: A Randomized Trial of the Effect of Vitamins E and C on 3-Year Progression of Carotid Atherosclerosis." *Journal of Internal Medicine* 248 (2000): 377–86.

Slavin, J. "Why Whole Grains Are Protective: Biological Mechanisms." *Proceedings of the Nutrition Society* 62, no. 1 (February 2003): 129–34.

Stephens, N. G., A. Parsons, P. M. Schofield, F. Kelly, K. Cheeseman, and M. J. Mitchinson. "Randomized Controlled Trial of Vitamin E in Patients with Coronary Disease: Cambridge Heart Antioxidant Study (CHAOS)." *Lancet* 347 (1996): 781–86.

Chapter 7: Conception Accomplished: Preparing for Pregnancy

Allen, L. H. "Multiple Micronutrients in Pregnancy and Lactation: An Overview." *American Journal of Clinical Nutrition* 81, no. 5 (May 2005): 1206S–1212S.

National Institute of Child Health and Human Development, National Institute of Health, nichd.nih.gov.

The National Women's Health Information Center, 4woman.gov.

Index